Long-term Care, Globalization, and Justice

Long-term Care, Globalization, and Justice

LISA A. ECKENWILER

The Johns Hopkins University Press

Baltimore

© 2012 The Johns Hopkins University Press
All rights reserved. Published 2012
Printed in the United States of America on acid-free paper
9 8 7 6 5 4 3 2 1

The Johns Hopkins University Press
2715 North Charles Street
Baltimore, Maryland 21218-4363
www.press.jhu.edu

Library of Congress Cataloging-in-Publication Data

Eckenwiler, Lisa A., 1967–
    Long-term care, globalization, and justice / Lisa A. Eckenwiler.
        p.   ;   cm.
    Includes bibliographical references and index.
    ISBN-13: 978-1-4214-0550-6 (hdbk. : alk. paper)
    ISBN-10: 1-4214-0550-4 (hdbk. : alk. paper)
    ISBN-13: 978-1-4214-0551-3 (electronic)
    ISBN-10: 1-4214-0551-2 (electronic)
    I. Title.
    [DNLM: 1. Long-Term Care—ethics—United States. 2. Aged—United States.
3. Internationality—United States. 4. Public Policy—United States. 5. Social Justice
—United States. 6. Socioeconomic Factors—United States. 7. World Health.
WT 31]
    362.16—dc23   2011034761

A catalog record for this book is available from the British Library.

*Special discounts are available for bulk purchases of this book. For
more information, please contact Special Sales at 410-516-6936 or
specialsales@press.jhu.edu.*

The Johns Hopkins University Press uses environmentally friendly book
materials, including recycled text paper that is composed of at least 30 percent
post-consumer waste, whenever possible.

For Thom

Contents

Acknowledgments

I owe thanks, first of all, to the Center for American Progress for offering me a fellowship in 2006 that enabled me to begin the necessary research for this project. Special appreciation goes to Jonathan Moreno and Sam Berger for their generous support. I am also grateful to le Centre de Recherche en Éthique à l'Université de Montréal, especially Ryoa Chung, Daniel Weinstock, and Martin Blanchard, for a fellowship in the summer of 2008, which allowed me to further my investigation of the global justice literature and to lay the foundations for the book.

For opportunities to present the work at various stages I offer thanks to the organizers and participants of: the Health in an Unequal World research network, especially Ted Schrecker and Ronald Labonté; the National Citizens' Coalition for Nursing Home Reform's 2007 annual meeting; the Manchester Workshop in Political Theory and Public Health in 2008; the On Lok annual meeting in 2008; the International Journal of Feminist Approaches to Bioethics (IJFAB) conference in 2008; the 2009 meeting at the University of Ottawa on the Migration of Health Professionals; the workshop on Care Labor Migration and Global Justice held at the Canadian Conference on International Health in 2009; and the workshop on Global Justice and Health Inequalities at the International Studies Association in 2011. Certain people warrant particular mention: Angus Dawson, Rebecca Shaw, Mary Rawlinson, Ivy Lynn Bourgeault, Rosie Tong, Lisa Forman, Andrea Kalfoglou, Bruce Jennings, Christine Straehle, Donald Redfoot, Jim Nelson, David Concepción, Judy Feder, and Henry Claypool. For research assistance, I am indebted to Zainab Ashraf, and Bonnie Gomolka.

My most heartfelt gratitude goes to my mom and my steadfast friends, especially Manuela, Suzanne, Kristine, Ryoa, Mira, Mary, Jean-Michel and Hermes, Steve and Zoubeida, Ashby, Angela, Barb, Angus, and Béatrice. Above all, I owe love and thanks to my grandmother, her caregivers and their families, and to Thom.

Long-term Care, Globalization, and Justice

Introduction

I wish I could remember her exact words. "Don't cry honey," urged one of my grandmother's regular evening caregivers when I came back to her room from the hospital. "It will keep her spirit from passin'" . . . or something close to that. Later that day, the night aide who had called at 4 a.m. to tell me they had taken her to the hospital, told me everything that happened before the emergency medical technicians arrived and while they were there.

I had persuaded my grandmother—the brightest star in my childhood galaxy—to move to be near us. I arranged for and coordinated her care, took her to doctors' appointments and emergency rooms, visited her every few days and talked with her every night, and spent the day spooning with her as she died. Yet these caregivers —one Jamaican and one African American—were the women who did the daily work of caring for her.

This book comes from reflection on the connections between elderly grandmothers and mothers in places like Boston, Los Angeles, New York, and Washington, DC, to others in Kingston, Port au Prince, Manila, and Kerala, and patients, like those living with HIV/AIDS; between daughters and granddaughters in the United States to those here from the Philippines and Haiti. These connections, forged from the policies and practices of government officials, international bankers, health care executives and human resource personnel, recruiters, employers, and the choices of individuals, tend to be obscured in discussions of long-term care policy, yet they raise complex and pressing questions of responsibility.

Thanks in part to a century of progress in public health and medicine, many people are enjoying longer lives. These changing demographics are generating a greater need for long-term care. In the United States alone, the number of people using nursing facilities, alternative residential care, or home care services is expected to increase from roughly 15 million to 27 million in 2050 (U.S. DHHS and DOL 2003). Yet by all accounts, long-term care is "no longer viable" (Miller, Booth, and Mor 2008, 450). Moreover, experts argue, we are "without an abiding social purpose that we as a society buy into collectively" (451).

What Levine, Albert, Hokenstadt, et al. (2006, 305) refer to as the long-standing absence of a "comprehensive, coherent, long-term care public policy" clearly raises profound concerns for the burgeoning population of dependent elderly. This policy void generates problems for family caregivers, who find themselves navigating perilous terrain as they strive to support their loved ones and often suffer ill health themselves. It also threatens long-term care workers, who are born and trained in the United States but find themselves working and living in low-resource conditions. At the same time it has serious implications for the health care workforce and those in need of care in the global South, in countries that are themselves burdened by aging populations, chronic conditions, and, often, HIV and AIDS. As governments in affluent countries confront "growing *demands and expectations*" [my emphasis] for affordable, quality long-term care services (OECD 2005, 10), health workers, including nurses and paraprofessionals, are migrating from countries in Africa and the Caribbean, from the Philippines, India, China, and South Korea at unprecedented rates to take up positions in long-term care. A recent report argues that the growing reliance on migrant care workers is a symptom of inadequate long-term care policy (International Oranization for Migration 2010, 7).

Indeed, atop a long list of worries U.S. experts cite inadequate workforce and family caregiving capacity (Institute of Medicine

2008; Miller, Booth, and Mor 2008); yet many so-called "source countries" have even more rapidly growing long-term care needs and higher burdens of disease, and at the same time suffer from lower care-worker-to-population ratios than do destination countries like the United States (Weinberger 2007). The state of long-term care policy in the United States is contributing, however indirectly and unintentionally, to global workforce shortages and deepening health inequalities, and, indeed, to what some describe as a global "crisis in health" (WHO 2006a). The central message from the recently convened Global Forum on Human Resources is that workforce shortages in low- and middle-income countries, many of which serve U.S. long-term care needs, are "one of the most pressing issues of our times," given the implications for global health inequalities (Chatterjee 2010).

This book explores the global landscape of care work; that is, the organization and structure of care, specifically long-term care, in the context of globalization and its implications for justice and health equity. Here I invoke a not-so-novel epistemological framework, ecological thinking, and demonstrate its value not only for understanding relationships between "wind and water, food chains, soil drainage and rock formation . . . and animal and plant susceptibilities" (Code 2006, 40) but also for guiding long-term care policy; that is, for understanding and responding to the ethical and policy issues involved in long-term care work, paid and unpaid, as it is organized globally. Ecologist Rachel Carson emphasized interdependence among species and traced "patterns of chemical damage and natural fragility-vulnerability across a range of interrelated ecosystems" (47); here, I trace the dense—and increasingly transnational—connections that organize and constitute long-term care, highlight sites of vulnerability, and explore responsibilities to the dependent elderly, their caregivers, and populations in source countries. I hope to show that ecological thinking can guide long-term care planning by understanding and ethically assessing the interdependence among particular policy sectors (health, economic, labor, and immigration); places (long-term care settings in the affluent global North and health care settings in the global South, homes, and workplaces, and the "transnational space" in which policy decisions are made, operationalized, and carried out and in which emigrants live and move); and people (the dependent elderly and family caregivers in the United States, paid care workers, including emigrants, and those with needs for care living in the countries that serve U.S. markets). I argue that an ecological analysis enables policy makers to see how the existing state of long-term care policy generates injustice—injustice that is global in scope—and, prospectively, can help address this through an innovative theory of global health equity and coordinated, comprehensive policy recommendations.

What, then, first, do I mean by ecological thinking?

Defining an Ecological Approach

As typically understood, ecology describes "the study of patterns in nature, of how those patterns came to be, how they change in space in time, why some are more fragile than others" (Kingsland 1995, 1). Ecology, as a discipline, though, is diverse. Population ecology describes the study of "the interrelationships between organisms and their surroundings" (Pickett, Kolasa, and Jones 2007, 12), or "the processes influencing the distribution and abundance of organisms, the interactions among organisms, and the interactions between organisms and the transformation and flux of energy and matter" (Institute for Ecosystem Studies n.d.). Ecosystem ecology involves "the study of ecological systems, and their relationship with each other and with their environment" (Pickett, Kolasa, and Jones 2007, 12). Ecosocial theories in epidemiology "seek to integrate social and biological reasoning . . . to develop new insights into determinants of population distributions of disease and social inequalities in health." They investigate "who and what is responsible for population patterns of health, disease, and well-being, as manifested in present, past, and changing social inequalities in health" (Krieger 2001). Philosophers who embrace ecological thinking explore the interrelationships between the environment, social and political relations, technological and informatic structures, and our embodied agency and subjectivity (Genosko 2009). The focus here is on how these structures and relations constitute our corporeality, shape the way we experience spatiality, and exercise agency. How, they ask, do we as embodied, interdependent, embedded beings navigate particular terrains from day to day, survive, and, ideally, flourish (Grosz 1995; 1999; and 2005)?

The greatest inspiration here comes from the work of Lorraine Code (2006). Ecological thinking, on her account, "proposes a way of engaging—if not all at once—with the implications of patterns, places, and the interconnections of lives and events in and across the human and nonhuman world" (4). An ecological analysis situates knowledge generation and, in turn, policy making—efforts in particular places populated by particular people and conceived as intersecting "with other locations and their occupants" (Code 2006, 21). By revealing the links between particular "ecosystems" (here, long-term care settings in the affluent North and health care settings in the global South, homes and workplaces, and "transnational space"), policies, and people, ecological thinking is concerned with "imagining, crafting, articulating, and endeavoring to enact principles of ideal cohabitation" (24). Stated differently, it aims to "discern conditions for mutually sustaining lives within a specific locality, be it an institution of knowledge production, an urban setting, a workplace, a geographical region, a community, society, state or *the interrelations among them*" [my emphasis] (60–61).[1]

Ecological thinking has four distinctive elements. First, this epistemological framework is critical of and aspires to replace reductionist models that "isolate parts of nature [and/or social life] so as to obscure the constitutive functions of multiple and complex interconnections" in generating effects (Code 2006, 42).

Second, thinking ecologically highlights broad patterns as well as particularities among people and places. "In its commitment to complexity, [this approach to knowing] urges attention to detail, to minutia, to what precisely—however apparently small—distinguishes this patient . . . from that, this practice, this locality from that, as Rachel Carson would distinguish this plant, this species, from that . . . all the while acknowledging and respecting their commonalities, where pertinent" (Code 2006, 280). By paying keen attention to local particulars, Code argues, ecological thinking aspires to "generate responsible re-mappings across wider, heterogeneous . . . terrains" (50).

Third, ecological thinking is attuned to power relations. It situates its investigations "within wider patterns of power and privilege, oppression and victimization, scarcity and plenty" (Code 2006, 280). Above all, it seeks to resist and, ultimately, to replace "ecologically uninformed policies of mastery that commonly filter evaluations of multiple forms of 'damage' through utilitarian assumptions about the end (= greater productivity, efficiency, and human comfort or safety) [whose?] justifying the means (= the conquest of nature [and human others]" and aims "critical-constructive analysis . . . at the entitlements and presumptions endorsed by governing conceptions of security and enhancement, at the evaluative ordering of species [and peoples] built into patterns of justifying these purposes, and at the overarching picture of the world—the dominant social imaginary—that holds this conceptual apparatus in place" (12).[2]

Finally, ecological thinking invokes a longer temporal and spatial view, across terrains and timeframes, and so allows for identifying effects and their sources that may not be readily apparent and for envisioning interventions that can be sustained over time.

Consider, as Code (2006) does, Rachel Carson's critique of conventional studies on the effects of pesticides:

Viewed vertically, from a top-down observation position that draws linear, causal connections from chemical applications to the destruction of a targeted pest, the power of the then-new post–World War II chemicals to rid the environment, efficiently, of such diseases and insects . . . [seems] impressive. Yet viewed horizontally, taking a longer temporal and spatial view, across terrains and time-frames where their effects become manifest more slowly, the chemicals do not merely obliterate a predetermined target species. . . . They also contribute to the destruction and/or sterilization of insect-eating birds, ground squirrels, muskrats, rabbits, domestic cats, sheep and cattle, destruction that often does not follow the spraying instantaneously. (45)

In having the capacity to take the long view, ecological thinking can be understood as emphasizing the future over the past and present. The stakes here are high. As Elizabeth Grosz argues, unless we develop concepts of time and duration that "welcome and privilege the future, we will remain closed to understanding the complex processes of *becoming* [my emphasis] that engender and constitute both life and matter" (Grosz 1999, 16).

Ecological Thinking, Long-term Care Work, and Global Justice

Thinking ecologically about long-term care in the context of globalization yields a different picture than one generated by a reductionist focus on one of many singular issues related to long-term care that have received varying degrees of attention. These include the bleak conditions that often characterize long-term care for the elderly, even in affluent parts of the world; the implications for the elderly of the way that health care services are structured; the implications for family caregivers of efforts to contain health care costs; the struggles of family caregivers working in the paid labor force; the working conditions of paid caregivers in the United States and other affluent countries; the emigration of health workers; and the global shortage of health workers such as nurses. As these issues are understood and discussed, the relationships among them tend to be obscured.

To be fair, some scholars have acknowledged relationships between many of the concerns here. For instance, the relationship between working conditions in health care and long-standing problems with recruitment and retention of nurses and direct care workers has been a focus of attention (Stone and Wiener 2001). Similarly, some have analyzed the relationship between working conditions and quality of care (Paraprofessional Health Institute 2011). Others have examined the implications for families of cost containment and fragmentation in health care (Levine 1998; 1999; Stone 2000; Nelson 2002). There are many discussions of the nursing shortage in affluent countries, these countries' growing reliance on foreign-educated nurses, and the deepening of health inequalities (Chen, Evans, Anand, et al. 2004; Chaguturu and Vallabheneni 2005; Kingma 2006; WHO 2006a; 2006c). Relationships between the high-level professionals who have benefited from economic globalization and the serving classes who support them as maids and nannies have been highlighted (Sassen 2002a; 2002b). Literature on the international division of reproductive labor has offered insights on transnational families, especially the effects on children of the feminization of emigrant labor (Hochschild 2000; Parreñas 2005). On the whole, however, conversations have not fully reckoned with the relationships between policies and stakeholders in the global context of long-term care. For instance, the relationships between the elderly, family caregivers, and health and labor policy; between the elderly, family caregivers, and global economic and immigration policy; between the elderly, family caregivers, long-term care workforce planning failures, and populations in parts of the global South where health care systems are fragile; and between the elderly, family caregivers, economic, immigration, and labor policy, and social reproduction in the global South.

There have been gestures in the direction I want to go. Aimed at engaging with the "interconnectivity" of long-term care concerns, the National Commission for Quality Long-term Care (NCQLTC) stipulates that "efforts to reform long-term care require an ... integrated approach" (NCQLTC 2007, 18). They rightly link the workplace and family caregivers in their analysis, yet they give no attention to labor policy—specifically policy on family leave—or to the growing global interdependence of the long-term care work-force. A World Health Organization (WHO) committee argues for developing services that "evolve over time, and adapt to changing national conditions"; that respond to the "pattern and pace of increases in long-term care needs as they are affected by epidemiological phenomena, and the availability of family support"; and that are "integrated into the overall health and social policy framework of each country" (WHO 2002c, 55). This comes closer, yet it still suggests that efforts ought to be organized at the national level (see also OECD 2005). To the extent that discussions are framed in nationalist, or statist, terms, they obscure global connections and, in particular, the rapidly growing structure of interdependence that characterizes the provision of long-term care.

Plan of the Present Work

The first part of this book offers an ecological analysis of care work.[3] Taking inspiration from Carson and Code, I move "transversely across geographical and social landscapes" (Code 2006, 7), incorporating literature from global health and health care, economics, development and postcolonial studies, geography, feminist theory, and moral philosophy to explore the plight of the elderly and their caregivers. In chapter 1, I describe changing demographics and the growing need for long-term care in the United States and go on to identify the present policies and practices that undermine the quality of care for the dependent elderly; consideration of long-term care in countries other than the United States is beyond the scope of my project. From there, I examine the plight of unpaid caregivers, specifically family members who provide assistance, and consider the set of policies and practices that threaten them as a group and that also put pressure on care labor markets.

In chapter 2, "The Plight of Paid Workers in Long-term Care," I examine the processes and structures that shape the lives of those working to care for the dependent elderly for pay, identifying the historical and current sociopolitical and economic factors that contribute to their plight. I concentrate for the most part on nurses and direct care workers, such as nurse aides, home care aides, and personal care assistants.[4] These workers may be the most essential members of the global health workforce, serving as the principal providers of basic health services as well as long-term and palliative care (Fleming, Evans, and Chutka 2003; Priester and Reinardy 2003; WHO 2003). The first part of the chapter focuses on nurses and other care workers who have been educated in the United States. I then turn to consideration of why those educated in low- and middle-income countries emigrate to the United States, which is now the largest importer of nurses and other care workers (Aiken 2007; Dumont and Zurn 2007). I focus on the United States' primary source countries and regions for long-term care: the Philippines, the Caribbean, and, increasingly, India. I refer both to migrants and emigrants, and to the extent possible I distinguish between them. I am most concerned about emigrants here; that is, those who leave one country to live in another.

In chapter 3 I argue that an ecological approach helps to demonstrate that, all told, care work is organized transnationally—through economic, labor, immigration, and health policies established primarily by governments, international lending bodies, transnational corporations, and other for-profit entities—in such a way that it creates and sustains injustice against the dependent elderly and those who care for them and weakens the care capacities of countries and their health systems, particularly those of source countries. Although we might describe the harm done in a number of ways—for instance, in terms of threats to welfare, constraints upon agency and autonomy, the denial of equal moral worth, or the unfair distribution of resources—the best way of understanding it is in terms of structural injustice.

In chapter 4, "An Ecological Ethic," I explore how responsibilities to address harm—specifically, structural injustice—flow from the nature of the relationships between governments, international lending bodies, the for-profit sector, and the other agents who contribute to the global organization of long-term care work. The grounding of responsibility, I argue, can be found not merely in shared humanity, compassion, or participation in the processes that generate injustice but also in our nature as ecological subjects who are interdependent and, indeed, constitutive of one another. The social connections, even "across distance" as they are often framed, are even tighter between us than most theorizing about justice acknowledges. The focus of justice on this view, moreover, shifts from individuals toward ecological subjects, situated temporally, spatially, and socially, who need particular kinds of habitats in which to become and endure. Taking a page from the work of geographers, I propose that we understand responsibility in long-term care as a matter of "ethical place-making" (Raghuram 2009); moreover, I suggest that perhaps this should apply to global health equity more generally. When it comes to long-term care in a global context, our responsibilities are to avoid creating conditions of deprivation that threaten people's capacities for becoming and enduring and to support conditions that nurture and sustain becoming and enduring.

Finally, chapter 5 offers recommendations for policy and practice, specifically for how, with the benefit of an ecological approach, policy makers, planners, and families can come to organize long-term care policy and planning efforts around ideals of justice and sustainability.

As a final point of introduction, I want to bring attention to the problem of what allows for some kind of "closure" on an ecological analysis. My aim with this project is, above all, to highlight the myopia of analyses to date concerning what is relevant to ethical long-term care policy and planning and their temporal constraints and to begin to address these serious, even life-threatening, liabilities by proposing a conception of justice to guide future thinking and action. My effort here surely suffers from limitations on both counts. No doubt there are relevant issues I have not addressed. We might wonder, for instance, whether climate change is contributing to care worker emigration and to growing needs for long-term care around the world. It is also not impossible that decades from now the health and long-term care systems of source countries, and in turn the health of their populations, will be better than what will be seen in today's wealthiest countries. I have highlighted what seem to be, given available evidence and our limited powers of thought, the most salient factors that shape long-term care in a global context, both currently and in at least the mid- if not long-range future. A hallmark of ecological thinking is humility; this work emerges with all that is due.

CHAPTER ONE

The Plight of the Dependent Elderly and Their Families

The past several decades have seen significant improvement in the health of older adults. In the United States and many other parts of the world, people are living longer and with less chronic disability than ever before (WHO 2003; Federal Interagency Forum on Aging Related Statistics 2006). The aging population is burgeoning. While currently the proportion of older persons is 17 percent, by 2050 it is expected to be 26 percent (Weinberger 2007, 17). In the United States in particular, between 2000 and 2050 the population age 65–74 will grow from 18 million to 35 million, the population age 75–85 will grow from 12 million to 26 million, and most dramatically, the population age 85 and above—the fastest growing segment of the population—is expected to quadruple, growing from 4 million to 21 million (U.S. Census Bureau 2008).

While there has been considerable debate concerning the nature and extent of future long-term care needs, especially given declining rates of disability in recent decades, the consensus is that they will grow (Institute of Medicine 2008).[1] Even though many people over 65 are in good health, the great majority—as many as 80 percent—of older adults contend with at least one chronic disease (hypertension, heart disease, and arthritis, for instance) that calls for care over time (Wolff, Starfield, and Anderson 2002; Pleis and Lethbride-

Cejku 2007). Many suffer from two or more (Anderson and Horvath 2002, 2004). Many struggle with "geriatric syndromes" or conditions that tend not to fit into specific disease categories, such as: depression, sensory impairment, incontinence, malnutrition, and osteoporosis (Cigolle, Langa, Kabeto, et al. 2007; Inouye, Studenski, Tinetti, et al. 2007). A significant number are diagnosed with mental health conditions ranging from mild mood disorders to depression to severe cognitive impairment (U.S. Administration on Aging 2001; Johnson and Wiener 2006). An estimated 42 percent of those over 85 have Alzheimer's disease (Alzheimer's Association 2007). The elderly are more vulnerable to injury and acute illness as well. There are, not surprisingly, important differences across various demographic categories and subgroups (Institute of Medicine 2008). Marked increases in the age and disability levels of many care recipients are likely to lead to a greater demand for paid care workers given that the care needed may be increasingly complex and require a higher level of skill than many family caregivers, historically the first line of care for the elderly, can provide (U.S. DHHS 2000; Wolff and Kasper 2006; Kramarow, Lubitz, Lentzner, et al. 2007).

A Growing Problem

According to The Urban Institute's Retirement Project, even under the most optimistic scenario the size of the older adult population in need of assistance will grow significantly. At best, they argue, by 2040 "the number of older adults using paid home care will increase by three-fourths . . . and the number in nursing homes will increase by two thirds. Over the same period, the number receiving help from their adult children will increase by about one third" (Johnson, Toohey, and Wiener 2007, 3). The aged population will be more diverse than ever before, as well, with declining numbers of whites and increases in the percentage of Blacks, Hispanics and Asians (de Voelker 2010). These changing demographics—attributable to lower mortality and greater control over reproduction—

give rise to a growing need for long-term care, defined as the "wide array of medical, social, personal, and supportive and specialized housing services needed by individuals who have lost some capacity for self-care because of a chronic illness or disabling condition" (U.S. Special Committee on Aging 2000).

Meanwhile, if we look globally, we see that population aging is a worldwide phenomenon, affecting all regions and most countries (Weinberger 2007). As noted above, by 2050, the population aged 60 and above worldwide will have more than tripled from 600 million in 2000 to 2 billion, moving from 17 percent of the population to as much as 26 percent. The oldest old, or those eighty and above, will increase from being just 1.4 percent of the population to 4.3 percent. Projections further suggest that elderly populations in many low- and middle-income countries are growing more rapidly than those in affluent ones (Shrestha 2000; WHO 2003). Nearly 250 million of the approximately 420 million people over sixty-five live in developing countries, and expectations are that the majority will live there in coming decades—especially in sub-Saharan Africa, Latin America, the Middle Eastern crescent, Asia and the Pacific Islands, as well as China and India (WHO 2002a). Compared to wealthier countries, these mostly low and middle-income countries will undergo this demographic shift quite quickly, even as they continue to contend with the burden of diseases like HIV/AIDS and tuberculosis, and with considerably less in the way of resources, including human resources (WHO 2002c; Weinberger 2007).

But to return for now to the United States, what lies behind the claim that long-term care "is no longer viable" (Miller, Booth, and Mor, 2008, 450)? What, more precisely, explains the dilapidated state of long-term care, which imperils many of the elderly, leaves most bereft, and creates poor, even harrowing, conditions for their caregivers?[2]

The Sorry State of Long-term Care

Inadequate Capacity

As noted at the outset, long-term care experts cite inadequate workforce and family caregiving capacity as their top concern (OECD 2005; Institute of Medicine 2008; Miller, Booth, and Mor 2008). Despite current conditions and the rapidly rising need in the United States and many other countries, a persistent shortage in the pool of paid caregivers is expected to grow, and the capacity of the "informal" support system (i.e., family and other unpaid caregivers) is expected to diminish. I elaborate on these points below and in Chapter 2, but the point to emphasize here is that what some have called a "care crisis" is facing the United States and many other countries (Stone and Wiener 2001; Harmuth 2002; Paraprofessional Health Institute 2003; WHO 2006b).

Institutional Dysfunction

Most of those who need it live at home or in community settings (Agency for Healthcare Research and Quality 2000), but the institutions that provide long-term care are a focal point for concern. In the 1980s worries about nursing home quality culminated in the 1987 Omnibus Budget Reconciliation Act (OBRA), which raised standards and enhanced regulation. While OBRA did generate improvements, the institutions that exist to provide long-term care to the dependent elderly—nursing homes, alternative residential care, including assisted living facilities, which is the fastest-growing form of long-term care for older adults (Maas and Buckwalter 2006), and adult day care centers—continue to be plagued by a lack of funding, and poor and even unsafe conditions. Facilities, especially for-profit nursing homes, continue to be cited frequently for violations that bring harm—physical, and other—to residents (U.S. GAO 2005; U.S. Administration on Aging 2007; Commodore, Devereux, Zhou, et al. 2009). One study found that in 2007, a breathtaking 94 percent of for-profit nursing homes (who have the biggest market share) were cited for violations of health and safety standards (Pear 2008). Ninety-one percent of government nursing homes were cited, as were 88 percent of nonprofit homes. Approximately 17 percent had deficiencies that caused "actual harm or immediate jeopardy" to residents. The problem is even worse than we know: officials responsible for evaluating nursing homes reportedly frequently overlook major deficiencies (Pear 2006).

More generally, critics target "the oppressive, regimented life of traditional institutional environments entrenched in the biomedical model, which are organized to facilitate the efficient delivery of care while treating elders primarily as clinical entities and downplaying psychosocial and spiritual needs as well as overall quality of life" (Miller, Booth, and Mor 2008, 456). Long-term care institutions, they argue, "too often warehouse people, [are] terribly inflexible, and [do not] provide anything like a home." (456). Maybe most telling are the remarks of the former head of a large nursing home chain, Beverly Enterprises, a previous PepsiCo executive: "There really are an enormous amount of similarities between this and the world I came from [namely, Taco Bell]" (Abelson 2002).

Inadequate Training

Health care for the elderly is, more often than not, provided by professionals and other health care workers with little or no special training in geriatrics or long-term care (Institute of Medicine 2008). In 2007, just over 7,000 physicians were certified in geriatric medicine. The specialty suffers from a lack of prestige—indeed, many top students are actively discouraged from pursuing it—and very low compensation in comparison to others (Association of Directors of Geriatric Academic Programs 2004). In each year from 2007 to 2009 fewer than 100 graduates from U.S. medical schools went on to take up postdoctoral training in geriatrics (American Geriatrics Society 2009). Estimates are that by 2030, there will be only one geriatrician for every 2000 elderly people.

As for nurses, the vast majority of baccalaureate programs have no courses in geriatrics. While over 50 masters programs prepare advance practice geriatric nurses, the average program has five students. Combined they graduate approximately 300 students annually. In all, less than 1 percent of the nation's RNs are certified in the specialty (Reinhard and Young 2009). Management practices of nurses in leadership positions and working as frontline supervisors have been clearly demonstrated to play a crucial role in ensuring quality care, yet few receive formal training for such opportunities (Reinhard and Reinhard 2006).

As for direct care workers, or "paraprofessionals"—nursing aides or nurse assistants, home health aides, and personal and home care aides, the primary providers of paid care for the elderly—training is either minimal or altogether lacking. Seventy-five hours of training are required for home health aides and nursing assistants working for home health agencies or in nursing homes, and there are no federal requirements for workers hired directly by the elderly or their family members or those who work for agencies providing "unskilled" home services (Paraprofessional Health Institute 2003; Direct Care Alliance 2005; Gross 2007).

Fragmentation of Care

The lack of integration, or even cooperation, between different kinds of care—assorted specialties, and acute and long-term care—is a source of great concern for the elderly (Eaton 2002; Kane 2003). Even though most have several conditions that call for attention, health care is structured in a highly fragmented way, lacking cohesive, inclusive, team-oriented relationships among sub-specialties (WHO 2003). And as older adults move from one type of care setting to another—say from hospital to long-term care—there is often little or no coordination among providers (Parry, Coleman, Smith, et al. 2003; Boockvar, Fishman, Kyriacou, et al. 2004; Foust, Naylor, Boling, et al. 2005; Levine, Albert, Hokenstad, et al. 2006; Levenson and Saffel 2007).

Payment systems are also fragmented, which leads to inefficient and inadequate care (MedPac 2006a and 2006b). Designed to respond to needs for acute care—while appropriate at its inception—Medicare is poorly suited to address the ongoing care demanded by chronic conditions (Brown, Peikes, Chen, et al. 2007). Despite the fact that patients tend to see many different providers at many different sites of care, Medicare offers no payment for communication and coordination among providers (Guterman 2007). Medicare also fails to pay for services provided by nonphysicians, except in rare circumstances (Lawlor 2007). Medicaid pays for long-term care for the poor and for the most part requires people to be indigent. Despite the strong preference for community-based care, it is biased toward institutions. For people eligible for both programs, that is, the most vulnerable older adults, "the lack of coordination between the programs often results in inefficiencies and fragmented services" (Institute of Medicine 2008, 23). In short, different eligibility rules, incentives, and measures of success contribute to "schismatic care" (Kane 2003, 81). These payment systems also have a relatively short time horizon: nursing home payments are calculated on a daily basis, and for post-hospital home care, prospective payments create an incentive to get out quickly. They thus ignore the long-term nature of needs, and perversely, given the way payment is structured, "the unstated incentive is to create or maintain disability" (ibid.).

The trend in long-term care since the 1980s has been toward decentralization, privatization, and informalization (Harrington and Pollock 1998). State and local governments, in other words, have come to take on the responsibilities of managing long-term care, and services have come to be provided more often in the home, increasingly by for-profit organizations, along with family caregivers.

Ageism

What underlies much of the failure described here is no doubt the spectre of ageism—spawn from a set of blinkered ideas that emphasize self-reliant subjects and ignore the significance of care and dependency relations in human life (Biggs and Powell 2001; Nelson 2002; Alliance for Aging Research 2003). When it comes to health care, this not only can cause harm to the identities and self-respect of the elderly, it also affects both the amount and the quality of care they receive. Assumptions that they are confused and noncompliant, and even unworthy recipients of health care resources further undermine their care (Asch, Kerr, Joan, et al. 2006).

The Plight of Family Caregivers

Our shared and inevitable human dependency generates a need for care. Care, according to the understanding I will follow here, is "a species activity that includes everything we do to maintain, continue, and repair 'our world' so that we can live in it as well as possible. That world includes our bodies, our selves, and our environment, all of which we seek to interweave in a complex, life-sustaining web" (Fisher and Tronto 1990, 40). Without care, infants and children cannot develop their capacities, and adults, even healthy ones, but certainly the ill, the old, and the disabled, can struggle to thrive. For the dependent elderly, care is crucial to maintaining many capacities, and as with children, can be necessary for survival. Care, it is essential to add, is not only a concern for the ill, infirm and injured; even the most robust require a vast array of care services and support. Care, in sum, provides the foundation for the survival, and under ideal conditions, flourishing of all people and is especially vital for the most fragile among us.

Of course, care is not merely valuable to individuals. It generates "fundamental public goods" (Ogden, Esim, and Grown 2006, 333). Without care labor, societies could not develop or prosper. Indeed, "care produces goods with social externalities. . . . It creates human and social capital—the next generation, workers with human and social skills who can be relied on, who are good citizens" (Folbre 1999, 80) and sustains us over the course of life, especially during infancy, illness, disability, and decline. The work of caregivers, those who help to provide for the personal and/or health needs of others who are dependent is, thus, at the core of social organization and reproduction. Whether moved by desire, a sense of obligation, fear of reliance on paid care, cost, or some combination, around the world family members are the primary providers of care, including long-term care for the elderly. Indeed, most people in need of care—roughly 80 percent—receive it solely from so-called "informal" caregivers, including family members, friends, neighbors and others (Wiener 2003; Pan American Health Organization 2004b; Johnson and Wiener 2006; International Longevity Center and Schmieding Center for Senior Health and Education Taskforce 2007). Even when they are not the primary caregivers, family caregivers still provide substantial support and assistance.

At least 30 percent of adults in the United States serve in this crucial capacity (AARP 2008). While it varies greatly, on average family members offer as many as 25 hours weekly (National Alliance for Caregiving and AARP 2004). The average is 200 hours of support per month, more than a typical full-time job (Johnson and Wiener 2006). The evidence that their efforts benefit the elderly in the United States is clear and abundant (Miller and Weissert 2000; Picone, Wilson and Chou 2003; Yoo, Bhattacharya, McDonald, et al. 2004; Mittelman, Haley, Clay, et al. 2006). Adult daughters provide the most care, in terms of the variety of care provided and the amount of time spent, doing everything from serving as a source of emotional support, coordinating care, accompanying the elderly to medical appointments, managing finances, and often delivering medical care (Pan American Health Organization 2004b; Wolff and Kasper 2006; International Longevity Center and Schmieding Center for Senior Health and Education Taskforce 2007; Johnson, Toohey, and Wiener 2007; Wolff 2007; AARP International 2008). On the whole, the work of family caregivers—the vast majority of whom are women—"represents a critical piece of the global health workforce that is poorly documented and understood" (WHO 2006b; Skjold 2007, 16).

The profile of families, however, with decreases in the numbers of adult children, growing participation of women in the paid workforce, and geographic dispersion, is adding to the challenges of ensuring adequate long-term care (Stone 2000; Bachu and O'Connell 2001; Fleming, Evans, and Chutka, 2003). Indeed, like the care workforce, the numbers of available family caregivers are not keeping pace with the growth of the long-term care population. As the demands on them grow, family caregivers, to put it charitably, have little in the way of recognition or support.

The Social and Economic Value of Caregiving

The care provided within families lacks social standing and garners little respect in many countries, and is not typically seen as work, or in economic terms, as productive (Folbre 1999; Folbre 2001). What this ignores, of course, is that "any person's public existence floats upon the enormous amount of care work and reproductive labor that has come before and transformed a human infant into a capable citizen" (Tronto 2006, 4), or that is sustaining an aging, yet still enduring person. Care, put differently, "is the deep and ignored background to citizenship" (4), and more broadly, to economic and social flourishing.

Feminist economists and theorists of the gendered social relations of production have noted that while this work is discounted by standard economic theories that exclude things produced in the household as opposed to the market, and that ignore the transfer of value from the household to the market, caregiving labor makes a fundamental contribution or "input" into the processes of production. Yet societies are highly invested in the gendered and unequal division of such labor for it leads to surpluses and savings in public expenditures (Badgett and Folbre 1999). Those who have tried to attach a dollar figure suggest that in the United States alone, the estimated worth of care work is somewhere over $375 billion, and on the rise (Arno 2006; National Family Caregivers Association and Family Caregiver Alliance 2006; Gibson and Hauser 2007; AARP 2008).

In a shift from earlier eras, the majority—more than half—of family caregivers in the United States and other high-income countries are employed in the paid labor force (Kovner, Mezey, and Harrington 2002; Johnson and Wiener 2006). But for the most part their employers offer scant support. While this phenomenon holds true in many other countries (WHO 2003), the United States is distinctive in having some of the weakest family leave policies in the world (Heyman, Earle, and Hayes 2007; Pavalko, Henderson, and Cott 2008). Roughly eight percent of private sector employers provide paid family leave, and most often it supports the best-educated and white, but not blue collar, workers (Congressional Research Service 2009).[3]

Beyond what employers make available in the United States, the federal Family and Medical Leave Act (FMLA), enacted in 1993, promises workers up to twelve weeks of unpaid leave in any twelve-month period to care for a baby, ill child, spouse, parent, or for oneself. It is quite limited in only covering businesses with 50 or more workers, those who have worked for a given employer for a least one year. This leaves many workers—over half—uncovered, and studies show that even for those who are eligible, it doesn't offer adequate support for most families, particularly working class ones (Waldfogel 2001; Williams and Boushey 2010). Changes made in 2008 to the FMLA have been subject to criticism for making leave even harder to obtain, and for punishing workers and violating their privacy when they do take leave (National Partnership for Women and Families 2007).

While the FMLA has arguably generated benefits for family caregivers and those for whom they care, as many as 78 percent of workers, especially those at lower income levels, say they cannot afford to take unpaid leave (AFL CIO n.d.). At the same time, many workers worry that if they use leave they will risk losing their jobs or being seen as unreliable. The Center for Worklife Law found that legal complaints by workers alleging discrimination based on their status as caregivers (called family responsibility discrimination) increased approximately 400 percent in the ten-year period from 1995 to 2005 (Center for Worklife Law 2008). Given this disconnect between the workplace and the workforce, the United States has been described as having "the most family-hostile public policy in the developed world" (Williams and Boushey 2010, 1).

Health Policy and Practices
Fragmentation

The lack of integration, or even cooperation, between different kinds of care—assorted specialties of medical care and long-term care—is not only a problem for the elderly. It is also a major problem for their caregivers. This, coupled with the fact that most health professionals have no training in elder care, compounds the work and stress of unpaid caregivers who must learn how to navigate the system in order to ensure that their loved ones get the professional services they need (Levine 1998; Levine 1999; Donelan, Hill, Hoffman, et al. 2002).

Another problem concerns the fragmentation between institutional care and home care, and thus between paid and unpaid caregivers, with family members struggling to understand the "system" and providing care themselves for which they feel unprepared (Weuve, Boult, and Morishita, 2000; Levine, Albert, Hokenstad, et al. 2006; Weinberg, Lusenhop, Gittell, et al. 2007). Many health professionals working in hospitals tend to overlook the fact that families have different capacities to provide for the needs of their elderly, dependent members. Yet rather than provide comprehensive evaluation and pay attention to the particular circumstances of families, like the availability of a dedicated caregiver, financial assets, housing situation, communication and decision-making skills, surrounding social network, etc, as it relates to the kind and amount of care needed, existing health care system policies and practices (like discharge planning) make only rough assessments of families' particular capacities to provide care out of the hospital.

Similarly, in home care, despite the fact that for many people family members and home care workers are inextricably linked, among advocates and policy makers, family caregiving and paid care work in the home tend to be seen as separate worlds, with independent policy agendas competing for attention and resources (Better Jobs Better Care 2005). Overall, public and institutional policies tend to focus only (and not always keenly) on the individuals in need of care and not those around them providing it (Wiener 2003).

Cost-cutting and Underinvestment

As many governments restructure their roles to spend less on health and social needs, and health care institutions cut costs, a "care gap" has emerged that ultimately relies upon family care-givers to contribute additional energy and resources. In the past decade, efforts to contain explosive health care costs have included shortened stays in hospital settings, and early discharge of patients. The success of this strategy hinges upon the availability of family members—women—to serve as home care providers, or what has been described as a sort of "semi voluntary conscription of unpaid health care workers, who generally lack any professional training for their tasks" (Nelson 2002, 278; Donelan, Hill, Hoffman, et al. 2002; Wolff and Kasper 2006). At the same time, arguing on the basis of cost-effectiveness and consumer self-determination, choice, and benefit, many governments have begun to move toward restructuring their role in the providing of care and welfare servic-es—especially home care and personal care assistance—and in the process, shifted responsibilities onto family members (Jenson and Jacobzone 2000; OECD 2005; Christopherson 2006; Ogden Esim, and Grown 2006). While it goes by other names in other countries, "consumer-directed care" in the United States involves giving cash to the dependent to purchase care, typically in their own homes. The "Money Follows the Person" initiative relocates people from nursing homes, for example, while "Choices for Independence" aims at avoiding nursing homes altogether and providing people who need long-term care services assistance at home (Kassner, Reinhard, Fox-Given, et al. 2008).[4]

The trend in many places, including the United States, is toward informalization and privatization. As Nicola Yeates (2009) explains: "These reforms have amounted to processes of privatization insofar as they involve policies infusing for-profit providers into . . . care delivery systems with the voluntary and state sectors providing care for . . . low-income long-term dependent populations. They also amount to the informalisation of care provision, based on achieving reduced state expenditure costs by reducing the unit costs of labour, with the transfer of a large portion of provision of long term . . . care to women" (30). But again, most women in high-income countries are employed in the paid labor force and lack adequate support from public policy or their employers.

Even as family members do most of the needed care work, over a quarter of the elderly have some combination of unpaid and paid help, a trend that appears to be on the rise (Federal Interagency Forum on Aging Related Statistics 2006). Recognition of the plight of family caregivers led to the passage in 2000 of the National Family Caregiver Support Program (NFCSP), under the Older Americans Act, providing funding for states to assist family and other "informal" caregivers, counseling and training, and respite care.[5] Nevertheless, rising demand and a dearth of support—due to a confluence of social, economic, health, and labor policies and practices enacted by government and others—increase their reliance on paid care workers. A growing number of these care workers are women from countries plagued by their own unmet and growing needs for care (Polverini and Lamura 2004; Van Eyck 2004; Seavey 2007; Uhlenberg and Cheuk 2008). In the next chapter, I begin to explore this concern.

CHAPTER TWO

The Plight of Paid Workers in Long-term Care

The 500,000 registered nurses (RNs) and licensed practical nurses (LPNs) now working in long-term care in the United States provide direct care as well as care coordination and supervision in high and mid-level management positions (Reinhard and Young 2009). Direct care workers, however, play the most integral role in long-term care, providing up to eight out of every ten hours, or 70 to 80 percent, of paid care for those who are elderly, disabled, and/or suffer from chronic conditions. In 2006, there were more than 3 million direct care workers (Paraprofessional Health Institute 2011). These care workers, also known as paraprofessionals, are employed in a variety of settings. Only 17 percent can be found in hospitals; the rest are in long-term care settings: nursing homes, assisted living facilities, and individual residences (Paraprofessional Health Institute 2011).

Depending upon where they work, direct care workers perform a wide range of tasks, including providing assistance with mobility, bathing, dressing, toileting, cooking, eating, housekeeping, shopping, transportation, and with paying bills. Like nursing, this work is highly gendered. Nearly 90 percent of direct care workers are women. More than half are non-white or Hispanic. The field, indeed, is sometimes described as a "minority industry," for the percentage of minority workers is significantly higher than in the U.S. workforce as a whole (Montgomery, Holley, Deichert, et al. 2005; Wolff and Kasper 2006; Paraprofessional Health Institute 2011).

Home health and personal care aides have been identified as being among the fastest-growing occupational groups (U.S. Bureau of Labor Statistics 2007; Paraprofessional Health Institute 2010a). Demand for direct care workers in home settings, already their most common place of employment, is expected to increase for several reasons. Cost containment in health care, the growing complexity and cost of long-term care, and the diminished capacity of family caregivers to meet elders' needs may all increase the demand. Additionally, as states continue to respond to the U.S. Supreme Court's 1999 decision, *Olmstead v. LC*, which held that people with disabilities must receive services in noninstitutional settings whenever possible, the need for such workers will expand. A growing number of them are hired on the gray market (Martin, Lowell, Gozdziak, et al. 2009).

While the importance of nurses and direct care workers is indisputable and on the rise, they face a difficult plight.

Social Values and Health Policies

Around the world, paid care work generally suffers from a poor public image and a lack of social respect (Folbre 2001; Kittay 2001; Miller, Booth, and Mor 2008). Those who care for pay also confront difficult working conditions. Nurses in the United States point to such problems as underinvestment in the health sector, staffing that is insufficient to support quality patient care, increasing hours on the job, rotation between units, centralized decision making that denies them participation (including participation in decision making regarding patient care), inadequate opportunity for continuing education and professional development, and poor compensation (Heinrich 2001; Berliner and Ginzberg 2002; Steinbrook 2002; Institute of Medicine 2003). Many, though by no means all, of these concerns can be attributed to health care restructuring in the United States that was carried out in the 1990s under the rubric of "managed care." Aimed at "improving efficiency" and reducing costs, managed care called for reducing staffing levels and substituting nurses with less training—such as LPNs and nurse aides—for RNs (Halford, Savage, and Witz 1997; Norrish and Rundall 2001; Weinberg 2003). Frustration with poor working conditions and low morale, in part because of such restructuring measures, are concerns cited by nurses around the world (Allan and Larsen 2003; Gordon 2005; Royal College of Nursing 2007).

These problems described by nurses are exponentially greater for direct care workers (Paraprofessional Health Institute 2011). This sector of the health workforce reports high rates of job stress and low satisfaction, even when they recognize the importance of their work (Stacey 2005; Brannon, Barry, Kemper, et al. 2007; Castle, Engberg, Anderson, et al. 2007; McGilton, Hall, and Wodchis et al. 2007). Regarded as "unskilled," direct care workers enjoy little if any respect in society or in the settings where they work (Bowers, Esmond, and Jacobson 2003; Better Jobs Better Care 2007). Home care aides, in particular, are officially regarded as "companions" rather than workers. This was laid down by a 1975 federal labor regulation and upheld by a 2007 U.S. Supreme Court decision (*Long Island Care at Home, Ltd. v. Coke*). As a result, those who employ such workers are not required to pay minimum wage or to provide overtime pay as required by the Fair Labor Standards Act.

Direct care workers as a group tend to be employed in the most underresourced settings and to earn very low wages (Paraprofessional Health Institute 2010b). In 2009, the median hourly wage for direct care workers was $10.58, significantly less than the median wage for all U.S. workers, $15.95. Using the U.S. Census definition, approximately 15 percent are poor; two out of every five rely on public benefits such as food stamps and Medicaid (Paraprofessional Health Institute 2011).

Not only does this group of care workers make extremely low wages, but many of them, especially home health aides, also lack benefits, including health insurance and sick leave (Better Jobs Better Care 2004; Paraprofessional Health Institute 2011). Nearly 30 percent go without health insurance. This may be attributable to several things, either singly or in combination: direct care workers may be hired privately by families who cannot offer health insurance, they may work for a small employer who does not offer it, or they may be unable to afford the premiums and copayments when employer-sponsored coverage is available. Perversely, however, direct care workers have higher than average rates of diabetes, asthma, and other chronic conditions and have one of the highest rates of job-related injury among all occupations (Newcomer and Scherzer 2006; U.S. Bureau of Labor Statistics 2009). Most of their injuries are sustained as a direct result of their efforts in caring for patients. They also often lack retirement benefits, which can, over time, keep them in an economically perilous position (Paraprofessional Health Institute 2011).

Tellingly, the former Taco Bell/PepsiCo executive, later a nursing home executive, quoted in chapter 1 notes: "Taco Bell competes with Beverly for these people" (Abelson 2002). As experts in long-term care argue, indeed, "many people who are working in long-term care are devalued, treated as criminals and paid extremely low wages" (Miller, Booth, and Mor 2008, 455).

Such conditions are in no small part responsible for the severe care worker shortage—what some call a "care crisis"—facing the United States (Stone and Wiener 2001). Nursing and direct care work is now characterized by unprecedented vacancies and turnover rates, with a declining number of people entering the field, retention problems, and a growing trend toward early retirement. Turnover rates among nurses in long-term care are currently over 50 percent (National Commission on Nursing Workforce for Long-Term Care 2005). For direct care workers, rates are breathtakingly high: 40 to 60 percent of home health aides leave a job after less than a year, and 80 to 90 percent leave within two years (Paraprofessional Health Institute 2011). For direct care workers in assisted living facilities, the average turnover rate per year is 42 percent

(Maas and Buckwalter 2006). In nursing homes, turnover is, on average, 70 percent annually, and in some cases it even exceeds 100 percent per year (Decker, Gruhn, Matthews-Martin, et al. 2003; Stearns and D'Arcy 2008). More than 90 percent of nursing homes report insufficient staff to provide even basic, much less optimal, care (Lawlor 2007). Estimates are that the country will need between 3.8 million and 4.6 million nurses, nurse aides, home health, and personal care workers by 2050 in order to meet the coming demand, an increase of 100 to 140 percent over 2000 levels (Scanlon 2001; U.S. DHHS HRSA, 2004a; U.S. DHHS HRSA 2004b; Gerson, Oliver, Gutierrez et al. 2005).

While these conditions might be addressed by any number of strategies, an increasingly popular one involves the employment of women from low- and middle-income countries in nursing and direct care positions, an endeavor that in some cases is preceded by targeted recruitment (Priester and Reinardy 2003; Chaguturu and Vallabhaneni 2005; Redfoot and Houser 2005). This strategy is part of a growing trend not just toward the informalization and privatization but also the globalization of long-term care (Holden 2002).

The Transnational Flow of Nurses and Other Care Workers

According to the Organization for Economic Cooperation and Development (OECD), "migration played a more important role in shaping the medical workforce over the last ten years than it has, on average, since the 1970s" (OECD 2008). Health worker migration is not a new phenomenon. In the postcolonial era, as many developing countries began to develop and expand their health services and to educate their citizens to staff them, some of their more educated workers left for wealthier countries, often, given language and other cultural ties, those of the colonists (Buchan, Parkin, and Sochalski, 2003; Choy 2003). The transnational flow, however, has never been higher (Dumont and Zurn 2007). Health workers are migrating at unprecedented rates. Part of the feminization of international migration, many women are seeking work abroad as nurses and other care workers (Ramirez, Domingues, and Morais 2005; Van Eyck 2005; Kingma 2006; Reichenbach 2007). The United States is currently the largest importer, and the only net receiver (Aiken 2007; Dumont and Zurn 2007; OECD 2008). While dispersed around the country, these workers are found in the greatest numbers in densely populated parts of California, New York, New Jersey, Florida, and Illinois.

Although the evidence is still limited, and what is available is hard to decipher for a host of reasons,[1] existing data, which focus on physician and nurse migration, reveal important trends. The percentage of foreign-trained nurses among new registered nurses has doubled since 1995, and for nearly a decade now, the number of foreign-trained nurses entering the U.S. labor market has increased at a rate faster than that of U.S.-educated new nurses (Cheung and Aiken 2006). Under managed care, not only did emigrant nurses take up many of the lower-level positions available, often despite advanced training, but when the market for nurses expanded again a few years later, emigrant nurses filled still more positions (Pond and McPake 2006). Economic trends do indeed fluctuate. As I write this, global recession has ebbed emigration. Still, the rising demand should cause this to shift yet again.

U.S. hospitals employ many of these foreign-educated nurses (American Hospital Association 2007), yet with the rise in the numbers of the dependent elderly, a growing number are finding employment in long-term care settings (Priester and Reinardy 2003; Xu and Kwak 2005; Redfoot and Houser 2005; Leutz 2007). An estimated 30 percent of foreign-educated RNs work in long-term care, and approximately 48 percent of RNs working in home care specifically come from abroad (U.S. DHHS HRSA 2004a; U.S. DHHS HRSA 2004b; Martin, Lowell, Gozdziak, et al. 2009). Among foreign-educated LPNs, up to 80 percent are employed in long-term care.

In 2008, the top countries sending nurses to the United States, as measured by the percentage of first time, foreign-trained candidates for the exam that grants licensure to nurses, the NCLEX, were the Philippines, India, South Korea, Canada, and Cuba (National Council of State Boards of Nursing 2008; Matsuno 2009).[2] For long-term care settings specifically, the top countries of origin for foreign-born nurses seem to be the Philippines, Jamaica, Haiti, India, and the United Kingdom (Redfoot and Houser 2005; Martin, Lowell, Gozdziak, et al. 2009). Notably, the presence of Chinese nurses in the United States has increased fourfold since 1995 (Dumont and Zurn 2007; Fang 2007).

A similar trend can be seen among direct care workers. Emigrant women are playing an increasingly integral role (Redfoot and Houser 2005; Leutz 2007; Browne and Braun 2008). Long a low-wage, "minority" industry, direct care work has become a transnational one. Approximately 20 percent of direct care workers are born outside the United States, most of them in low-income countries (Paraprofessional Health Institute 2011). Among home health aides, the foreign-born make up an estimated 24 percent, while they constitute 20 percent of nursing and psychiatric aides. Although the data are difficult to come by, the major countries of origin appear to be Jamaica, the Philippines, Mexico, Haiti, and certain African countries, including Nigeria and Ghana (Redfoot and Houser 2005; Martin, Lowell, Gozdziak, et al. 2009). The home care industry employs an especially high percentage of foreign-born workers, a trend that holds true for many countries. Women working in home care, notably, make the lowest wages among all direct care workers. They are more likely to be self-employed and hired privately by clients or their families (Montgomery, Holly, Deichert, et al. 2005; Seavey 2007). As noted earlier, a growing number of these home care workers are hired on the gray market (Martin, Lowell, Gozdziak, et al. 2009). Perhaps especially important is the point that foreign-trained care workers who emigrate to more prosperous parts of the world—namely, North America, Western Europe, and high-income countries in the Gulf and the Western Pacific—are increasingly likely to emigrate from low-income countries with a low supply of care workers and, in some cases, a high burden of disease (Dumont and Zurn 2007; Polsky, Ross, Brush, et al. 2007).

Along with the need for more care workers in the United States, a need generated to a great extent by policy choices, a complex configuration of other factors helps to facilitate this global flow.

Global Economic and Trade Policies

Underdevelopment in the global South and the emergence of neo-liberal economic policies may well be the greatest contributor to the modern-day movement of care workers around the world. With the aim of encouraging economic growth and promoting global economic integration and interdependence, international financial institutions, chiefly the World Bank and the International Monetary Fund (IMF) under the influence of dominant countries such as the United States, have compelled countries in the global South to balance budgets and become more competitive players in the global marketplace. Their main tools have been structural-adjustment policies, economic policies geared toward shrinking the public sector and expanding the private sector through, for instance, denationalizing state holdings, cutting public budgets for things like health care, education, childcare, and food, expanding the private sector and privatizing social services, welcoming foreign investment, and promoting exports, including exports of human capital (Moghadam 1999). In many places, structural-adjustment policies have led to reductions in employment, including health sector employment (Bach 2003; Buchan, Parkin, and Sochalski 2003; Stilwell, Diallo, Zurn, et al. 2004; Mackintosh and Koivusalo 2005), and caused many in the global South to seek work in richer nations in order to survive. More recently, the IMF's demand for ceilings on public wage spending has reportedly thwarted efforts to hire needed health workers and educators, even when funds are available (Schrecker 2008, 602).

The economic restructuring imposed on the global South has

affected women in distinct ways (Kuenyehia 1994). Many were employed in the public sector, not just in health care but also as teachers and administrative personnel, and so have been especially vulnerable to job cuts. Already the principal providers of care within families, reductions in health care and social services (reliant on women's availability) compel them to dedicate still more time to caring for the young, the elderly, and the ill (Dalla Costa and Dalla Costa 1995; Alcaron-Gonzalez and McKinley 1999). Even cuts in things like food and fuel subsidies disproportionately affect women in that they turn to less expensive and unrefined food products, which demand more preparation time.

Although many care workers emigrate for their own sake and that of their families given the economic conditions they confront, the governments of emigrants' home countries are also dependent upon them. Some have taken to recruiting their own citizens for care work abroad as part of their economic development plans. Emigrant care workers thus make substantial contributions not just to their own families but also to their home countries' economies (World Bank 2005; United Nations Population Fund 2006). Indeed, "an increasing number of . . . governments are beginning to view emigrants and their economic transfers as strategic resources to be 'captured' and incorporated in national development processes" (Ramirez, Dominguez, and Morais 2005; Sørenson 2005b, 1).

The Philippine government figures prominently in the political economy of emigration as the largest source of registered nurses working overseas (Go 2003; Lorenzo, Galvez-Tan, Icamina, et al. 2007). The country's complex migration infrastructure assesses global demands for Philippine labor, identifies labor shortages, works at generating demand for Philippine workers, and actively manages Philippine labor around the globe, including nurses. India and China, too, are coming to see human labor, including care work, as a valuable export (Fang 2007; Khadria 2007). The Caribbean, as well, has explored ways to profit from emigration (Sanders 2005).

The labor of women is especially vital under contemporary global economic policies and the industrialization processes they have spawned (Moghadam 1999; Pessar and Mahler 2003; Piper 2005; United Nations Population Fund 2006; Docquier, Lowell, and Marfouk 2008). While women's unpaid labor has contributed to global production, their presence in industries from textiles and electronics to pharmaceuticals, in the service sector, including health care, and in informal sectors of the economy has increased dramatically in the era of economic globalization. Women seeking care-based employment in more affluent countries as maids, nannies, nurses and paraprofessionals, as well as sex workers, have come to be an especially integral part of the global economy (Parreñas 2001a; Ehrenreich and Hochschild 2002; Kingma 2006). Current data show that highly skilled labor among women, including nursing, is rising especially quickly (Dumont, Martin, and Spielvogel 2007). Indeed, global economic policies have contributed to a modern-day transnational trade in care work, both skilled and so-called unskilled.

Free trade agreements, as well, have reduced trade barriers and contributed to job losses in the global South, thereby facilitating the mobility of people. Free trade blocs adopt measures aimed at encouraging the "free movement of labor," such as mutual recognition of qualifications or the easing of visa or permit requirements (Bach 2003, 27). "For key custodians of the global economy, including the World Trade Organization (WTO), the emigration of workers forms an integral and beneficial component of the globalization and the liberalization of the service sector" (Adlung 2002).

Immigration and Labor Policy in Host Countries

The U.S. Immigration and Nationality Act of 1965, also known as the Hart-Celler Act, represented a dramatic shift in U.S. policy. It abolished the national origins quota system that had been in place since the Immigration Act of 1924 and replaced it with a preference system that was more welcoming to people with skills in short supply and to those with ties to citizens or residents of the United

States. Nurses were among those considered highly desirable, and while Asians had been considered at the bottom of the list of desired entrants, they came in large numbers from former colonies like the Philippines in the wake of World War II (Le 2010).

In the context of contemporary economic globalization, selective immigration is increasingly used as an "instrument of industrial policy" (Ahmad 2005, 44). This is certainly true in the case of health workers, including nurses (OECD 2002; Buchan, Parkin, and Sochalski 2003). In the United States, H-1A visas were created for temporary employment of foreign-educated RNs under the 1989 Immigration Nursing Relief Act (Hoppe 2005). That program expired in 1996. Then in 1999, the Nursing Relief for Disadvantaged Areas Act established the H-1C visa for such nurses—500 per year—to work, for up to three years, in facilities facing staff shortages. It was reauthorized in 2005, but was then allowed to sunset at the end of 2009. The 2005 Emergency Supplemental Appropriations Act for Defense, the Global War on Terror, and the Tsunami Relief Act included provisions aimed at increasing the flow of foreign-educated nurses, allowing the U.S. State Department to release additional visas for nurses and physical therapists from the Philippines, China, and India and to reassign a designated number of EB-3 (employment-based) visas for countries—the Philippines, India, and China—that had reached their quotas. EB-3 visas are typically requested by employers with assurances to the Department of Labor that no U.S. workers are available and that current employees' wages and benefits will not be adversely affected by hiring workers from abroad. Notably, when seeking to hire nurses, no attestations are necessary (Arends-Kuenning 2006). An important route for nurses in supervisory and highly specialized positions is the H-1B visa, good for three years, with a possible three-year extension. Other legislative maneuvers have included the Emergency Nursing Supply Relief Act, which would remove the cap on the number of foreign-educated nurses and family members allowed into the country subject to a cap of 20,000 visas, and the proposed

Nursing Relief Act of 2009, aimed at creating a nonimmigrant visa for RNs.

Meanwhile, industry organizations in the United States (including the American Hospital Association, the American Health Care Association, and the National Center for Assisted Living), who regard international recruitment as a way to keep hiring costs down and improve retention, lobby for an easing of immigration requirements in order to gain access to nurses and other care workers (Buchan, Parkin, and Sochalski 2003; Pittman, Folsam, Bass, et al. 2007).

Direct care workers, by contrast, confront more challenges when it comes to emigration to the United States. No temporary visas are available for them, as the number of visas set aside for all less-skilled workers is currently capped at 5,000 per year (Leutz 2007). Some worry that the increasing demand and lack of legal avenues contributes to the illegal immigration of many women who end up working in long-term care, especially in the informal or gray economy in home care (International Organization for Migration 2005; Redfoot and Houser 2005). An estimated 21 percent of foreign-born direct care workers are unauthorized immigrants (Martin, Lowell, Gozdziak, et al. 2009).

The Recruitment Industry

While informal recruitment through social networks, including family members, former colleagues, and others, is an important piece of the migration story (Alonso-Garbayo and Maben 2009), the growing demand for care workers, especially nurses, has contributed to the dramatic growth in recent years of a for-profit international recruitment industry, involved in a range of activities related to recruitment, testing, credentialing, and immigration (Connell and Stilwell 2006; Pittman, Folsam, Bass, et al. 2007). In the late 1990s in the United States, there were roughly 30 to 40 companies engaged in international nurse recruitment, often operating on behalf of the health care industry. As of 2007, there were at least 270. Estimates are that 41 percent of foreign-born nurses working in the United States have been recruited from abroad.

Not only has the size of the industry surged, but so too has the number of countries in which recruiters operate (Van Eyck 2004; Pittman, Folsam, Bass, et al. 2007). In the early days of international nurse recruitment, there were roughly half a dozen countries. Now there are more than seventy, many of which have high burdens of disease and low nurse-to-population ratios. Based on available evidence, the industry is a lucrative one. Without these agencies and other employment promoters motivated by the potential for profit, analysts suggest, labor emigration would not be seen on such a massive scale (Kofman, Phizacklea, Raghuram, et al. 2000).

Gender Norms and Racial Stereotypes

The global division of long-term care labor is fueled by "the ideological construction of jobs and tasks in terms of notions of appropriate femininity ... *and* [my emphasis] racial and cultural stereotypes" (Mohanty 2003, 141). In the context of economic globalization, long-entrenched gender norms and attitudes about women's migration that might have precluded it have shown signs of shifting to allow for the possibility of participation in the global care labor force. Even in places where gender norms are firmly in place that assign women responsibilities for child-rearing, cooking, and caring for the home, women's mobility is increasingly acceptable for the sake of families' livelihood and, in particular, their financial well-being (Awumbila and Ardayfio-Schandorf 2008). Studies show a continuum when it comes to the influence of gender norms on women's decisions and perceptions concerning migration (Nowak 2009). Many see their role as helping to provide for the family, but they differ when it comes to their view on migration as a strategy. Some see their mobility as restricted, given what they count as costs of being away from their families; others, while taking family commitments equally seriously, see gender norms to be flexible in allowing them to migrate; and still others explicitly challenge gender roles, ranking their own professional opportunities higher than family obligations and rejecting the notion that they should rely on fathers or husbands financially.

I elaborate on the influence of racial and ethnic stereotypes below.

U.S. Labor Policies

The expansion of more affluent women's opportunities in the paid labor force within a context of scant employer support has generated employment opportunities for foreign-born women (Polverini and Lamura 2004; Van Eyck 2004; Bettio, Simonazzi, and Villa 2006; Kofman 2007). While there is tremendous variation among countries, the global trend is toward emigrant women serving for low wages as supplementary or principal care workers for the elderly (and children). "We see," as Saskia Sassen notes, "the return of the so-called serving classes . . . and these classes are largely made up of immigrant and migrant women" (Sassen 2002b, 258–59).

Women of color have for at least a century provided most of the care labor provided by nonfamily members in the United States. Evelyn Nakano Glenn's work (1992) examines the evolution of the racial division of reproductive labor, how it has "varied regionally and changed over time as capitalism has reorganized [it], shifting parts of it from the household to the market" (Glenn 1992, 3; Glenn 2006). Glenn documents how, as this labor came to be commodified, African American women in the South, Mexican American women in the Southwest, and Japanese American women in California and Hawaii at first served to relieve privileged white women of selected forms of household labor, including care labor, and eventually replaced them. Highlighting the racial division of labor within nursing and other paid care work, Glenn also explores the movement of women of color into lower-level positions in "public" reproductive labor; that is, sectors like health care and social services.

This analysis of the "hierarchy and interdependence among white women and women of color" (3) is illuminating for efforts to understand, in part at least, how direct care work became a minority industry. It also helps to shine light on the evolution of the importation of women from the global South, as capitalism and other structures reorganize care labor into a structural relationship based not only on gender, class, and race, but also citizenship (Parreñas 2000, 570). What we see now in long-term care, as Nicola Yeates argues, ought to be understood as a "contemporary expression of historically established arrangements . . . facilitated by advances in information and communication technology and shaped by contemporary organizational forms and dynamics of contemporary capitalist production" (Yeates 2009, 26). While paid care work has long been done by women of color, the modern commodification of care work tends now to take a transnational form (Bosniak 2009; Parreñas 2000). "Cheap and flexible, this model is [increasingly being embraced] to overcome the structural deficiencies of public family care provision [and workplace policy] and strikes a good balance between the conflicting needs of publicly supporting care of the elderly and controlling public expenditure" in privileged parts of the world (Bettio, Simonazzi, and Villa 2006, 282).

Source Countries in Particular

The Philippines

The Philippines is now the largest source of registered nurses working overseas (Go 2003; Lorenzo, Galvez-Tan, Icamina, et al. 2007). One estimate suggests that more than 70 percent of those who graduate each year leave for work abroad (Manzano 2005). In all, an estimated 85 percent of Filipino nurses work abroad (Brush and Sochalski 2007).

When asked why they leave, Philippine-trained nurses currently point to high and growing rates of unemployment in the Philippines and feelings of being "underutilized" even when employed (Lorenzo, Galvez-Tan, Icamina, et al. 2007). Many identify salary differentials as a primary reason for seeking work abroad. While in 2002, for example, the average annual salary for a nurse in the Philippines was between $2,000 and $2,400, in the United States the median salary for RNs was $48,900. They also cite desires for lower nurse-to-patient ratios, better working hours, and better opportunities for their own professional development and for their families' well-being (International Labour Organization 2006; Lorenzo, Galvez-Tan, Icamina, et al. 2007; Alonso-Garbayo and Maben 2009). Some also describe familial pressure: working abroad has come increasingly to be seen as an expected strategy for family survival, even a woman's duty (Ball 2000; Kelly and D'Addario 2008). This is not to suggest that all emigrant women come from the poorest families; many seem to be middle-class (International Labour Organization 2006).

Yet Filipino nurses have long been primed for emigration to the United States. Missionary and military involvement in the Philippines, along with targeted foreign-policy strategies, began fueling the mobility of Filipino nurses more than a century ago. As part of a broad effort to serve American colonists and military personnel stationed there with "modern" medicine, the Baptist Foreign Mission Society established the first nursing school in the country (the Iloilo Mission Hospital School of Nursing) in 1906 (Choy 2003). Many nurses were sent to the United States for additional training, sponsored by groups like Rockefeller, Daughters of the American Revolution, and the Catholic Scholarship Fund.

By the 1920s, though, efforts were well under way to export American-style nursing education and practice and bring "American professionalism, standardization, and efficiency" to the Philippines; that is, a "rational, scientific, and universalistic" approach (Brush 1995, 552). Funded in large part by the Rockefeller Foundation, the United States undertook "vigorous worldwide nursing and public health reform" as part of its broader internationalization efforts (Brush 1995, 542). Along with China and India, the Philippines was among the countries targeted (Healey 2006). Later, in the wake of World War II, in collaboration with the International Council of Nurses, Rockefeller introduced the Exchange Visitor Program to offer experience in American hospitals for nurses trained abroad, including those from the Philippines (Brush 1993; Brush and Sochalski 2007). By the mid-1960s, most were moving to jobs in U.S. hospitals (Brush 1995).

Since these early days, the numbers leaving have grown exponentially (Lorenzo, Galvez-Tan, Icamina, et al. 2007). The contemporary surge can be traced to the early 1970s, when, with the aim of developing what were to be temporary measures to ease unemployment, poverty, and the country's ailing financial system, President Ferdinand Marcos began to cultivate an explicitly export-oriented, debt-servicing development strategy. By the late 1990s, a complex, labor-exporting bureaucracy had emerged. With the passage of the Migrant Workers and Overseas Filipinos Act of 1995, the export of workers came to be administered by the Philippine Overseas Employment Agency (POEA), which assesses global demands for Philippine labor, identifies labor shortages, works at generating demand for Philippine workers, sets standards for overseas employment contracts, regulates the now-robust private recruitment industry, and actively manages Philippine labor, including nurses, around the globe (Lorenzo, Galvez-Tan, Icamina, et al. 2007; Jones 2008). At the same time, the Overseas Workers Welfare Administration (OWWA) provides such services as predeparture orientations, life and medical insurance, and offers scholarships. The Office of the Undersecretary for Migrant Workers' Affairs also supports workers abroad by providing legal assistance when needed and even medical and psychosocial aid. Nurse export forms an integral part of this institutionalized economic strategy. A small percentage of these emigrants are men; the majority are women. Since the 1980s, women labor emigrants have outnumbered men (Tyner 2004). By 2001, an estimated 72 percent of workers leaving were women, most of them trained as nurses (Philippine Overseas Employment Administration 2004). "At the end of the twentieth century, Philippine gendered labour migration and its diaspora have become the primary means for servicing Philippine indebtedness" (Barber 2000, 399).

Cultivating this care labor and its export are government-supported educational institutions, most in metro Manila (Palaganas 2010), that educate and train nurses, chiefly for foreign markets in Saudi Arabia, the United States, and the United Kingdom (International Labour Organization 2006). This training infrastructure has expanded exponentially over several decades to respond to a rise in other countries' recruitment efforts (Tan 2003). A first wave followed World War II; a second came in the 1970s; another came in the most recent decade. In the 1970s, the Philippines had approximately 80 nursing programs. As of 2005, as many as 450 nursing schools offered bachelor of science in nursing programs (International Labour Organization 2006). What is more, nursing schools here and in other low- and middle-income countries, are increasingly looking to U.S. universities to help with developing curricula and finding faculty to train nurses for export (Waldron 2004). Testing centers, too, have proliferated. So far, most are in Manila, yet they can be found sprouting in other provinces as well (Palaganas 2010). Private recruitment agencies now number more than 12,000, and in 2004 they had combined annual revenues of more than $400 million (Martin 2005).

Caribbean Countries

The Caribbean has one of the world's highest net-migration rates (United Nations 2002). While the greatest share of emigrants leave Guyana, Suriname, Jamaica, and St. Lucia, the major exporters of skilled labor in education and health care are Jamaica, Cuba, and Trinidad and Tobago. The United States, Canada, and the United Kingdom are the most likely destinations (Economic Commission for Latin America and the Caribbean 2006b). A shift away from an agricultural toward a service economy, increasing privatization, high unemployment, and declining growth in the wake of economic restructuring (structural adjustment was adopted in late 1970s), have contributed to the outward flow. An estimated 38 percent of the Caribbean population is poor.

Here, too, emigration for work has for centuries been an integral feature of the "character" of the population (Salmon, Yan, Hewitt, et al. 2007, 1355). The slave trade of the 18th and 19th centuries, post-Emancipation emigration, and the oil boom of the 1970s—when many went abroad for work in refineries—have all contributed to the "transnational households, livelihoods, and identities" that characterize the Caribbean (Thomas-Hope 2005, 53).

The emigration of nurses in particular can be traced back to the 19th century, when many left for education abroad with the intention of returning to help strengthen the region's health care system (Salmon, Yan, Hewitt, et al. 2007). Yet in the last decade, the numbers of workers leaving permanently for English-speaking destinations—especially women who are skilled professionals in education and health—have surged (Coward 2007). Estimates are that approximately two-thirds of the country's nurses have left, with roughly 400 per year migrating to the United States, Canada, and the United Kingdom (Economic Commission for Latin America and the Caribbean 2006a; 2006b). The reasons they cite are by now familiar: very low pay and inadequate benefits, feeling underutilized in relationship to education and skills (yet overworked, given staffing shortages), inadequate opportunity for professional development, inadequate involvement in decision making and support from supervisors, difficult working conditions, dissatisfaction with management and leadership, a lack of recognition and respect, and aggressive recruitment by employers in countries with shortages (Economic Commission for Latin America and the Caribbean 2003; United Nations Secretariat 2006; Yan 2006; Salmon, Yan, Hewitt, et al. 2007).

As part of a broader effort aimed at expanding business opportunities and strengthening economic relations, the region has established a single market economy (CARICOM). In keeping with this restructuring of the region's economy for the sake of greater competitiveness and poverty reduction, Mode 4 of the Global

Agreement on Trade in Services, or GATS, facilitates the movement of nurses out of the Caribbean, especially to markets in North America (Thomas, Hosein, and Yan 2005). While professionals like nurses and teachers are encouraged by host countries to stay, for the "unskilled" only temporary migration is encouraged. Home care and personal care aides, for example have access typically only to temporary employment (Brown 2008). Supporters argue for expanding both professional credentialing and occupational certification; indeed, they maintain that low- and middle-income countries have compelling interests in liberalization under Mode 4 (ibid.).

India

In the 1990s, India was in sixth place in the ranking of foreign-educated nurses seeking licensure in the United States. In 2004, with an emerging training, recruitment, and management structure, it was in second place (Khadria 2007). Between 1990 and 2000 the number of Indian RNs working abroad increased by 83 percent and the number of LPNs by 50 percent (Arends-Kuenning 2006). Kerala, which has well-educated women and high literacy rates, is the leading nurse-source region in India, producing more nurses than any other Indian state (Abraham 2004). Most of them come from the districts of Pathanamthitta, Kottayam, and Ernakulam (Thomas 2010).

Indian nurses say that income insecurity and poor working conditions in deteriorating sectors of the health care system lead them to leave. Many also point to a strong cultural disrespect of nurses given their association with the body and bodily fluids (Ramji 2002; Thomas 2006). Some scholars see a shift in the reasons for Indian women's emigration. While in the 1970s nurse emigration was a family strategy aimed at social mobility, the current pursuit of nursing among many is an actively pursued strategy that aims at increased autonomy and avoiding familial and other social expectations (DiCicco-Bloom 2004; Percot 2006).

Public and family attitudes in the state serve to support women's participation in the workforce. Most Indian nurses are Christian, which could be due to lower incomes among the Christian community and the attitudes held by some Hindus regarding nursing; namely, that it is polluting (Abraham 2004; Percot 2006). As in other source countries, there are (still understudied) regional differences with regard to emigration, and also variation among different religious and linguistic groups (Thomas 2006).

Whatever the modern motivation, nurse emigration has a long history linked to colonialism. The current export of nursing labor to English-speaking destinations like the United Kingdom and the United States might be traced back to the British Empire's Colonial Nursing Association. The association deployed nurses "lured by the seductions of empire, the spirit of adventure, and a newfound independence" to the colonies (Rafferty 2005, 13). Most Indian nurses graduate from government-sponsored schools, but private institutions are entering the field (Khadria 2007). As in the Philippines, nursing schools and training programs have proliferated. In 2002, 84 colleges of nursing reportedly offered BSc degrees. By 2006, there were 558.

Under neoliberal economic policies, this export is coming to be ever-bigger business (Healy 2006). Efforts are under way to reform nursing schools around international standards and the needs of importing countries and to become a major force of competition with the Philippines. Commercial recruiters play a prominent role in India's nurse-export economy. Targeting three geographic regions, New Delhi, Bangalore, and Kerala, especially Kochi, local for-profit recruitment companies, often in partnership with recruiters based elsewhere, now help to move Indian nurses abroad. With an eye on different labor markets, these agencies recruit nurses and offer assistance on licensing and visas.

At the same time, hospitals are joining the export industry through "business process outsourcing," or recruiting and training nurses for markets abroad for the sake of profit, perhaps as much as US$50,000 per nurse placed. Hospitals make deals with recruiting agencies, who screen and train nurses for positions abroad that offer salaries, benefits, in some cases housing and other assistance. Most activity so far has been in private-sector hospitals, but the government, too, is paying close attention (Khadria 2007). "It is a never-before-boom situation," according to the registrar of the Kerala State Medical Council (Nurse-ing [n.a.] 2003).

CHAPTER THREE

Tracing Injustice in Long-term Care

Explored from an ecological perspective, long-term care comes into view as a landscape made up of a set of interrelated, interdependent populations and habitats, all suffering under varying degrees of stress and strain, and some facing threats to survival. In this chapter I situate long-term care work in a global context and suggest that an ecological orientation helps to make clear the ways in which the configuration of political, economic, and other social and institutional structures—the "apparatus"[1] that transcends national boundaries and organizes long-term care labor—imperils the elderly and their caregivers and serves to deepen health disparities in less-privileged parts the world where care workers are scarce or absent altogether. By eroding conditions and capacities for care—especially (but not exclusively) in countries constituted to export care labor—over time it operates to sustain and reproduce spaces of deprivation.

I will go back and forth in discussing implications for family caregivers and paid care workers, but most of this chapter focuses on the plight of emigrant care workers. Following a general discussion of the implications for source countries, I consider the particular circumstances of the Philippines, the Caribbean, and India. I also explore possible consequences for the United States and other countries that draw on care labor from abroad.

Shaping the Subjectivities of Those Who Care

Seasoning

Many, maybe most, family caregivers desire to provide assistance to loved ones in need of long-term care; there is, however, good reason for concern about the caregivers themselves. There is now abundant evidence to suggest that care-giving responsibilities, doled out and taken on through gender norms and the social and institutional policies that exploit them, have profound effects on family caregivers, including effects on their sense of identity, agency, and self-worth (Nelson 2002). They report feelings of isolation and disrespect and a tendency to defer or even abandon their goals, both personal and professional (Levine 1999; Goldsteen, Abma, and Oesburg, et al. 2007).

The racial and cultural stereotypes at work in the global division of care labor help shape the identities of women who migrate and work in the paid care labor sector. Filippinas, for instance, are constructed as caring, obedient, meticulous workers and "sacrificing heroines" for their countries (Schwenken 2008); Caribbean women are seen as naturally warm-hearted and joyful; and Indian women as having "natural capacities" as carers (Abraham 2004). Such constructions serve the aims of governments, industry organizations, employers, and recruiters,[2] and even family caregivers in the North, yet they also perpetuate stereotypes and can constrain the imaginations and opportunities of women and girls (Brush and Vasupuram 2006; Rodriguez 2008).

Roland Tolentino's study of Filipinas' "integration into the circuits of transnationalism" (1996, 49) through the trade in mail-order brides provides an interesting comparison to care labor emigration. Both phenomena are "situated in the historical positioning of Filipina bodies into a transnational space inscribed in [gendered], colonial, militarist, and capitalist histories" (49) and involve their "packaging" and use as "a tool for (limited) economic empowerment" (53). In the same way that Filipinas are stereotyped and homogenized as "loyal, disciplined, and obedient" (Tyner 1996, 411), and their body parts—like their "nimble fingers"—idealized for work in the assembly lines spawned by the global economy, Filipinas are constructed as model export brides: "The preparation of the female [imagination and] body for work in multinational operations incipiently also prepares [them] for transnational work as a mail-order bride," argues Tolentino (1996, 55). With major capital at stake, governments in the global South have been "only too eager to provide this *habitat* [my emphasis]" for producing these subjectivities, determined by cost-benefit analyses to be valuable as export (53). And just as the Sears and Roebuck mail-order catalog—made possible by the expanding postal system's circulation of the colonies' products to the United States (63)—facilitated the emergence of the mail-order bride, the Web sites of contemporary nurse-recruitment agencies help to move nurses and other care workers from their homes in low- and middle-income countries into long-term care settings in the United States.

Overlapping varieties of nationalist rhetoric that support neoliberal economic policies operate in synergy with gender and racial stereotypes. One variety is organized around specific conceptions of national community and helps in compelling labor emigrants to organize their conduct around what is beneficial to states' economies (Raghuram 2009). "Like the new citizen-subject, the brain drain migrant is a particular subjectivity, forged by the needs of late capitalism." This subjectivity "is . . . constituted as an assemblage of morality and economic rationality," within which the migrant "acts in socially appropriate ways not because of force or coercion but because [her] choices align with . . . 'community interests'" (Ilcan, Oliver, and O'Connor 2007, 80). Other rhetoric emphasizes "the active citizen," a "reconfigured political identity . . . whose aim is to maximize . . . quality of life . . . by being [an] active agent in the market" (Schild 2007, 181). These rhetorical strategies, exalting capacities and even enforcing expectations for individual responsibility and choice, target poor women in specific ways, "encouraging and cultivating . . . forms of subjectivity that are congruent with capitalism in its latest phase" (199) (Fouron and Glick-Schiller 2001).

Women labor emigrants, however, find themselves in a bind. Although they are encouraged, even pressed—sometimes by governments, sometimes by family members, sometimes by both—to work and provide from abroad for their families and countries and are celebrated as "modern heroes," married women with children who do emigrate are often blamed for social ills such as divorce, poor school performance by children, and teen pregnancy in their home countries (Hochschild 2000; Sørenson 2005a; Parreñas 2006).

Flexibilization and Fragmentation

Along with these processes of being "seasoned"[3] as care laborers, women engaged in care work, especially those who emigrate, are subject to "flexibilization," a "process of self-constitution that correlates with, arises from, and resembles a mode of social organization" (Fraser 2009, 129; Fussel 2000). Its central features are fluidity, provisionality, and a temporal horizon of no long-term. This happens in a number of overlapping ways.

Family caregivers are compelled to navigate the fragmentation of the health care system, fill the care gap created by cost-cutting measures, and contend with the consequences of policymakers' division of family and paid care (Levine 1998; Cartier 2003). Those in the paid labor force typically find themselves distracted, distressed, working fewer hours, and taking unpaid leaves. Many pass up opportunities for advancement and retire early (MetLife, National Alliance for Caregiving, and the National Center on Women and Aging 1999; Pavalko and Henderson 2006; Lilly, Laporte, and Coyte 2007). Given "the temporally rigid way in which . . . professional commitments are defined today" (Hernes 2006, 313), family caregivers employed in the paid labor force are expected to be everflexible and contort themselves to make do.

For emigrant care laborers, transnational economic and other structures compel them to be mobile when most say they would rather work at home (Van Eyck 2004). Moving to labor markets in high-income countries—mobility that is allegedly upward and indisputably outward—may involve taking jobs below the education and skill level of care workers, a practice known as "downskilling" (Raghuram and Kofman 2004; Purkayastha 2005; Alonso-Garbayo and Maben 2009). There is also the rapid expansion of the informal or gray economy and the tendency under neoliberal economic policies to define more and more jobs as temporary and unskilled (Sassen 2002b), a phenomenon seen in care for the dependent elderly, especially at home.

As emigrant workers experience vertiginous upward and downward mobility to conform to labor markets, needed human health care resources go to waste.

Threats to Economic, Social, and Political Status

Not only are family caregivers often thwarted when it comes to career advancement, the reduction in work hours that they find is necessary often translates into a loss of economic and other benefits. Given the impact on pensions, Social Security, and other retirement savings vehicles, a substantial percentage of these caregivers are vulnerable to financial hardship and even poverty over time (Ettner 1995; Johnson and Lo Sasso 2006; Wakabayashi and Donato 2006). Minority caregivers, studies show, provide more care and are at greater risk for reduced work hours and lower incomes (McCann, Hebert, Beckett, et al. 2000; Covinsky, Eng, Lui, et al. 2001). As a group, family caregivers also often have considerable out-of-pocket expenses; some even deplete what savings they have in supporting family members' long-term care needs (Gross 2006c). One study found that 43 percent of employees worry about being able to provide for their parents (MetLife 2009). In all, "precariousness remains very high" (Jenson and Jacobzone 2000, 32).

At the same time, engaging in the work of care has implications for women's social and political positioning. As we saw in chapter 1, family caregivers tend to have little in the way of respect or social status. To the extent that they are defined by, or even associated with, the work of care, their status as citizens is diminished. Under a model of social organization that posits a rigid division between the public/private sphere, "citizenship is bestowed [only] on people for their public, not for their private, capacities" (Tronto 2006, 4).

Still, family caregivers in the United States and other destination countries fare far better than their sisters from the South. Their enhanced status as citizens, acquired to a great extent through increased participation in the paid labor force, has been supported by the labor of emigrant women who are more vulnerable socially and economically and who may themselves be denied a wider array of political rights (Bosniak 2009).

We can ask to what extent have initiatives aimed at supporting family and "informal" caregivers in the United States generated benefits. Studies are sparse, but one examination of the National Family Caregiver Support Program found that, while it facilitated the development of services and also expanded their range and scope, it allowed for "a great unevenness in services and service options . . . across the states and within states." The trend, one study found, is one of "local flexibility in service design, resulting in an inconsistent range of services and service options varying by locality . . . [and] gaps in caregiver services" (Feinberg and Newman 2006, 110).

The scant data on consumer-directed care reveal little effect on the gendered distribution of care work, labor-market participation, or women's often-fragile financial status:

> The benefits are presented as compensation for the costs incurred in caregiving, particularly when compared to a situation without benefit. However, they are sometimes offered at only symbolic levels and do not appear necessarily to minimize gender-related inequalities. (Jenson and Jacobzone 2000, 3)

Even in the best cases, it seems that payment covers little more than "the most basic needs of the elderly person or the caregiver" (27). What is more, critics maintain, the discourse of choice and self-determination around cash-for-care initiatives can obscure the gendered division of care labor in families and its implications for women's equality (Daly 2001).

With respect to emigrant care workers, although countries like the United States incentivize immigration for some skilled workers, including some categories of care workers, questions of immigration and citizenship are contested (Goldring 2001; Ball and Piper 2002; Ball 2004; Barber 2009; Dauvergne 2009). Care workers, especially the "unskilled," often lack citizenship in the countries where they are employed and therefore have a limited set of political rights (Deeb-Sossa and Mendez 2008; Bosniak 2009; Ong 2009). Countries "differentially incorporate" emigrants when it comes to immigration and citizenship status and freedom to negotiate contracts (Kofman and Raghuram 2006).

Due to immigration and travel laws that stringently control the entry and exit of some nationalities, some care workers are unable to travel home to visit (Schmalzbauer 2004). Many live in transnational families and engage in transnational care practices—that is, "extended family relations and obligations across space and time" (Hondagneu-Sotelo and Avila 1997; Baldock 2000, 221; Jones, Sharpe, and Sögren 2004; Parreñas 2005). Like other migrants who describe feelings of "dislocation" (Nynäs 2008; Pallasmaa 2008), some emigrant nurses describe the experience of "having a foot here, a foot there, and a foot nowhere" (DiCicco-Bloom 2004, 28; Van Eyck 2004). Notably, these harms faced by individuals can threaten relationships; they can lead others to "reinterpret our social or moral standing . . . [and] compromise the interpersonal bonds we have with them" (Miller 2009, 513).

As long-term care is provided in a context shaped by neoliberal economic policies and the denationalization of economies and renationalization of societies, emigrant women workers, especially those in low-wage lines of work, find themselves in a major bind:

they are constituted and constitute themselves to support the social and economic activities of the more privileged, often living in the destination country with diminished rights and protections and at the same time compromising their social and political status and participation in the home country (Parreñas 2001b; Escrivá 2004). Even nurses, the best-educated and best-employed of long-term care workers, describe both a sense of pride in their accomplishment and significant distress (George 2007). Especially troubling, though, is the plight of the growing number of undocumented noncitizen care workers, many of whom are working in the rapidly expanding field of home care (Meghani and Eckenwiler 2009). Often they are paid under the table; thus, labor laws may not be enforced and they are weakened in their ability to negotiate with their employers for fair wages and benefits (Browne and Braun 2008).

Women, especially Third World women, long-discounted as "valueless economic actors," are "crucial to building new economies and expanding existing ones" (Sassen 2002b, 255–56). On the one hand, there can be important gains for women who become wage earners (perhaps the primary ones) in areas like household decision making and expenditures, as well as in spatial mobility and even in the division of responsibility for child and elder care (Hondagneu-Sotelo 1994; Beneria 1999; McKay 2004; Pessar 2005). On the other hand, gender norms at home can restrict, even preclude, women's participation in decisions concerning how their remitted earnings are spent (Goldring 2003; Van Eyck 2004; 2005; George 2007; Kunz 2009; Lairap 2009), and to the extent that they are disproportionately engaged in forms of work designed to maximize profit for the architects of the global economy—low-wage, often temporary, part-time, casual, and home-based (Carr, Chen, and Tate 2000; Sassen 2002b)—prospects for greater equality under current conditions are at best uncertain.

Even as we recognize them as agents with capacities to create "new conditions and spaces for the re-working of . . . class, gender, and cultural identities" (Barber 2000, 399), an ecological perspective paints a picture of persistent vulnerability. Marilyn Frye's description of exploitation aptly describes the processes at work:[4]

> A tool is by nature or manufacture so constituted and shaped that it is suited to a user's interest in bringing about a certain sort of effect, and so its being put to use does not require its alteration. The case is otherwise with resources or materials; their uses or exploitations typically transform them. Trees become wood, which becomes pulp, which becomes paper. At each stage, the relations of the parts, the composition, and the condition of the thing used are significantly altered in or by the use. The parts and properties of the thing or stuff were not initially organized with reference to a certain purpose or telos; they are altered and rearranged so that they are organized with reference to that telos. A transforming manipulation is characteristic of this kind of using, of the exploitation of resources or materials. . . . Efficient exploitation of "human resources" requires that the structures that refer the others' actions to the exploiters' ends must extend beneath the victim's skin. The exploiter has to bring about the partial disintegration and re(mis)integration of the others' matter, parts, and properties so that as organized systems the exploited are oriented to some degree by habits, skills, schedules, values, and tastes to the exploiter's ends rather than as they would otherwise be, to ends of their own. In particular, the manipulations which adapt the exploited to a niche in another's economy must accomplish a great reduction of the victim's intolerance of coercion. (1983, 57–60)

Eroding Health

The health of care workers—paid and unpaid—is threatened by current arrangements in long-term care. Family caregivers are at heightened risk for chronic and elevated stress, poor physical health, depression, and death (Schulz and Beach 1999; Emanuel,

Fairclough, and Slutsman, et al. 2000; Cannuscio, Jones, Kawachi, et al 2002; Navaie-Waliser, Feldman, Gould, et al. 2002; Pinquart and Sørenson 2003; Vitaliano, Zhang, and Scanlan 2003; Christakis and Allison 2006; Messing and Östlin 2006; George 2007; Godfrey and Warshaw 2009; MetLife and University of Pittsburgh Institute on Aging 2010). Not surprisingly, here too important differences have been found among different groups of caregivers. Minority caregivers, for example, report worse health than whites and have higher rates of depression (Pinquart and Sørenson 2005). Poor health plagues women who care for family members around the world, indeed, not just in the United States (George 2007).

Those paid to provide care, especially direct care workers, report major physical and emotional strain and high stress, which leads in many cases to injury and/or poor health. This often goes unaddressed given the absence for many of health insurance coverage (Paraprofessional Health Institute 2011). Undocumented, noncitizen care workers are especially vulnerable (Meghani and Eckenwiler 2009). They generally cannot seek work in institutional settings that offer employer-sponsored health insurance. While many female citizen care workers do not have health insurance as part of their employment package, they might qualify for Medicaid. In contrast, all undocumented noncitizens were rendered ineligible for Medicaid by the 1996 "Illegal Immigration Reform and Immigrant Responsibility Act." That group is also not positioned to purchase health insurance because its members do not have Social Security numbers or sufficient financial resources. Moreover, deportation fears deter them from seeking care in public health clinics or emergency rooms.

Capital Gains for Source Countries?

For many source countries, the hope of government and other policymakers has been that remittances sent by those working abroad will serve to stimulate economic growth and development through investment and business opportunities, increased transfer of trade and knowledge, and over time reduce poverty (Domingues and Pos-tel-Vinay 2003; Kapur 2003; Connell and Brown 2004; Page and Plaza 2006). Migration can also generate "social remittances," or shifting "ideas, practices, identities . . . that affect family relations, gender roles, class and race identity," as well as social life more generally (Sørenson 2004, 4; McKay 2003). Some suggest that the very prospect of migration can nurture "human capital" by serving as an incentive for people to pursue education (Stark, Helmenstein, and Prskawetz 1998; Vidal 1998; Beine, Docquier, and Rapoport 2001; Connell and Brown 2004).

Remittances have not just grown steadily over the past decade, they have come to exceed the amount of official development aid, foreign private investment, and market capital flowing into source countries (Page and Plaza 2006). Since 1990, the rate of growth of remittances has seen a fivefold increase in low-income countries. The United States is currently the lead originator of remittances.[5] Some scholars have found that nurses are among the most reliable and generous remitters (Connell and Brown 2004).

While remittances indisputably channel billions of dollars in money and other goods, there is little consensus on the overall im-pact of migration on countries that export workers (Page and Pla-za 2006). Here I glean from a vast literature. Several studies have found that remittances contribute to economic growth and facili-tate production increases in agriculture, construction, manufactur-ing, and services, lead to greater entrepreneurial activity, and im-prove countries' access to international capital (Acosta, Calderon, Fajinzlber, et al. 2008). Others conclude that the effects are harmful and include, for instance, decreased labor-force participation and savings (Faini 2003; World Bank 2004; Chami, Fullenkamp, and Jahjah 2005; Bussolo and Medvedev 2007; Kim 2007). On poverty reduction, some evidence suggests that remittances do have a posi-tive impact (Adams 2004; Spatafora 2005; Page and Plaza 2006; Acosta, Calderon, Fajinzlber, et al. 2008; Gupta, Pattillo, and Wagh 2009). Some studies also have identified links between remittances and improvements in educational attainment (Rapoport and Docquier 2005). Still other studies have found that mothers in migrant households have more "health knowledge" than those in nonmigrant households (Hildebrandt and McKenzie 2006).

However, more recent research finds that skilled women's migration, now the fastest-growing kind of migration, significantly reduces overall welfare in poor source countries, as measured by adverse effects on infant mortality, under-five mortality, and secondary school enrollment (Dumont, Martin, and Spielvogel 2007; Docquier, Lowell, and Marfouk 2007; Nowak 2009). What is more, source countries can be harmed by losses in intellectual capital and, over time, innovation, national economic investment, and economic development (Lowell and Findlay 2002; Bach 2003; Buchan, Parkin, and Sochalski 2003; International Labour Organization 2006).

Worsening Global Health Inequalities

As debate persists on the ultimate impact of remittances, there is an overwhelming consensus that when health workers leave, population health erodes (Chen, Evans, Anand, et al. 2004; WHO 2006a; 2006c). Recent evidence suggests that the adverse effects of losing health workers are likely to be not compensated by remittances. This is because they do not contribute to the development of health systems or compensate for the economic losses of educated workers (OECD 2008).

According to the World Health Organization, 57 countries are facing a severe shortage of health workers (WHO 2006a; 2006b). These shortages serve to exacerbate global health inequities. More specifically, health worker shortages worsen inequalities in infant, child, and maternal health, vaccine coverage, and in response capacity for outbreaks, the consequences of conflict, and mental health care. Shortages in health personnel are said to be the most critical constraint in achieving the U.N. Millenium Development Goals and the WHO/UNAIDS 3 by 5 Initiative (Anand and Bärnignausen 2004; Chen, Evans, Anand, et al. 2004; International Council of

Nurses 2006). The loss of nurses and other care workers is especially troubling for they are the "backbone" of primary care in developing countries (Pan American Health Organization 2005; WHO 2006a; 2006c; Lynch, Lethola, and Ford 2008). Given their integral role in providing long-term care, these shortages also clearly present dire prospects for the rapidly rising population of elderly people and others with chronic and potentially fatal conditions like HIV/AIDS. Pressing demands on underresourced health care services, weakened by health-sector reform under structural-adjustment programs, indeed, are generating a crisis of care of colossal proportions. In some cases, shortages have led to a "virtual collapse" of health services in source countries (Packer, Labonté, and Runnels 2009, 214). The problem is so grave that the Joint Learning Initiative (2004) concluded that the fate of global health and development in the 21st century lies in ensuring the equitable management of human health resources. Echoing affirmation, the central message from the recently convened Global Forum on Human Resources is that workforce shortages in developing countries—many of which serve long-term U.S. care needs—are "one of the most pressing issues of our times," given their implications for global health inequalities (Chatterjee 2010).

There is wide variation among countries when it comes to the impact of health worker migration. If the workforce is small, numerically small numbers of migrating health workers can have profound effects (Gerein, Green, and Pearson 2006). Overall, however, the asymmetrical (that is, from low- to high-income) transnational transfer of care labor threatens to perpetuate and even worsen health inequalities—that is, health inequalities generally, but also in long-term care—to the extent that institutional and home care services are increasingly unavailable to support the chronically ill and the dependent elderly (*New York Times* 2003).

Where governments subsidize higher education, investments made in care workers can be effectively lost when they leave to work abroad or develop skills not applicable to their countries' needs and/or capacities. Another consequence is the stratification of health labor markets. The most-qualified workers are the ones most able to emigrate, yet as noted above in the mention of "down-skilling," they often take up jobs that call for skills below their formal training.

As in the global North, as populations age in developing countries, the public sector retreats and cost-containment strategies dominate the health sector, women then take on additional care responsibilities, including long-term care (Akintola 2004; Lopez-Ortega, Matarazzo, and Nigenda 2007; Harper, Aboderin, and Ruchieva 2008; Makina 2009). Governments facing underresourced health care systems have coped by "downloading" the burden of caring for those living with HIV and AIDS and others with long-term care needs onto women in communities and individual households, who often work without the benefit of formally organized health care services (Ogden, Esim, and Grown 2006; Wegelin-Schuringa 2006). Whether they stay home and care or emigrate and engage in transnational care practices, sometimes aided by family members in source countries with lesser economic prospects (Hochschild 2002), underresourced and eroding health care systems serve to further threaten women and compromise the health of those in need of care.

If we try to ascertain what are the specific effects on the countries that are main suppliers of care workers to the United States, we find that the best available data focus on nurses. Care workers with less training are largely underexamined.

Source Countries in Particular

The Philippines

Since at least the 1950s, following the Rockefeller initiatives— reportedly described by President McKinley as examples of "benevolent assimilation" (Brush 1995, 552)—Philippine nurses have been educated according to the standards of affluent countries. But the growing demand from abroad and widespread unemployment at home has led to the exponential expansion of a nursing education sector organized around the needs of nurses expected to leave (Lorenzo, Dela, Paraso, et al. 2005).

Emigrant Filippino care workers generally earn higher incomes for their families, gain personal and professional development opportunities, and often find greater independence (International Labour Organization 2006). Estimates are that Filipinas working overseas, including nurses, have come to remit more than US$8 billion annually (Ball 2008). Yet prepared to work in comparatively resource-rich hospitals and other health care institutions, they have on the whole become ill-equipped to address domestic needs, including long-term care.

Losing its skilled workforce "faster than it can replace them," Philippine health services are facing serious threats. With somewhere around 84 percent of employed nurses working abroad, and high numbers of physicians retraining as nurses for jobs abroad, the health system is highly vulnerable (Loreno, Galvez-Tan, Icamina, et al. 2007). As early as 1985, 47 percent of hospitals complained of being inadequately staffed, and extreme nurse-patient ratios existed. These poor ratios have been compounded by high staff turnover rates—as much as 60 to 80 percent per year (Ball 2008). Reports are that in some hospitals, the ratio of nurses to patients is as low as 1 to 60 (International Labour Organization 2006). Nurse-to-patient ratios are dangerously high in many rural areas (Lorenzo, Galvez-Tan, Icamina, et al. 2007). In all, nurse shortages in the country are at an estimated 6 percent and are expected to rise to 29 percent by 2020. Hospital closures and failures to meet standards for accreditation (which in turn affects reimbursement and financial viability) are among the signs of growing system inadequacies. Studies also describe serious stress and fatigue for those who stay (Lorenzo, Galvez-Tan, Icamina, et al. 2007). In sum, "the Philippine nurse education and labour market . . . has essentially become a training ground for overseas employers and the international trade in nurses, with potential longer-term consequences for [among other things] the Philippine health care sector and the quality of health care delivery" (Ball 2008, 340).[6]

According to the IMF, with remittances running at 13 percent of GDP, the Caribbean was the world's largest recipient of remittances. Although it is not clear that remittances are responsible, here, too, families and households who received them had higher incomes and lower poverty than others (Pienkos 2006). Analyses show, however, that remittances fail to compensate for the region's losses, especially in health and education (Richards 2005; Economic Commission for Latin America and the Caribbean 2006a; 2006b). The region has—along with the other challenges it faces—the second highest prevalence rate of HIV/AIDS after sub-Saharan Africa (Cock and Weiss 2000; CARICOM/Pan American Health Organization 2005). At the same time, the aging population is expanding rapidly, generating a growing demand for long-term, chronic care (CARICOM 2004; Economic Commission for Latin America and the Caribbean 2004; Vega 2007; Jones, Bifulco, and Gabe 2009; United Nations Population Fund-Caribbean n.d.). Yet due to emigration, the aged increasingly are unable to rely on their children for care, and health systems lack personnel.

Regionally, as many as 42 percent of nursing positions were vacant in 2005, especially in rural or remote areas (Salmon, Yan, Hewit, et al. 2007). Jamaica, for example, is facing a critical shortage of nurses. One estimate put the percentage of vacant positions in the country at 58 percent (Jamaican Ministry of Health 2004). Most countries have fewer than 30 nurses for every 10,000 inhabitants. Haiti, which has the region's biggest HIV burden, has 1.1 nurse for every 10,000 people (Pan American Health Organization 2005). Trinidad and Tobago lose an estimated one-third of the country's trained nurses to migration (Economic Commission for Latin America and the Caribbean 2003). As in the Philippines, the most highly trained and experienced nurses are the ones emigrating, leaving those with less training and experience to care for patients. Countries in the Caribbean do not have the educational capacity to replace these emigrants. According to one study, the cost to governments in the region of training for the roughly 400 nurses who leave each year is around $15 to 20 million per year (Economic Commission for Latin America and the Caribbean 2006a; 2006b). Jamaica has addressed this in part by recruiting nurses from other Caribbean countries (like Cuba and Guyana) and from India, Ghana, and Nigeria (Salmon, Yan, Hewit, et al. 2007). Shortages persist, however, threatening the quality of care and eroding working conditions for those who stay.

HIV/AIDS prevention programs, funded by external donors, cannot be staffed because doing so would take nurses away from the care of those already infected (Anderson and Isaacs 2007). Immunization coverage is also showing signs of weakening. Moreover, because some units in health care institutions have been compelled to merge, male and female patients are now more likely to receive care in the same unit, a situation that violates cultural norms (Pan American Health Organization 2005). Some countries in the region also show signs of weakening social support networks, which have been attributed in part to emigration (Pan American Health Organization 2004a, 2004b, and 2005).

Although Caribbean women who emigrate earn higher incomes abroad, studies also show that they can face considerable distress where gender norms tend to hold them responsible for family flourishing (Sørenson 2005a; Jones 2008; Jones, Bifulco, and Gabe 2009). Studies also suggest that older women may be affected by taking on the care of emigrant laborers' children (Pan American Health Organization 2004d).[7]

India

Less has been written to date about the impact of care worker migration upon India, but the country currently does not have enough nurses to meet its needs. The country has high rates of HIV/AIDS and other infectious and parasitic diseases, as well as rapid population aging, especially among poor, rural women (Gokhale 2007; Khadria 2007). India has among the lowest nurse-to-population ratios of all source countries; it also has the highest number of un-filled positions.[8]

The Erosion of Social and Political Capacity

By separating families, the transnational transfer of long-term care labor not only threatens health, and in some cases survival, in source countries, it stands to erode the very foundation of so-cial life. Given that the care done within families generates public goods and contributes to citizens' development and duration, when a country exports care labor it is exporting a society's capacities for social relations and reproduction (Truong 1996; Parreñas 2000). It is not just women's paid labor but also their unpaid care labor that is transferred out of source countries to stand in for what was once the unpaid care labor of other, now more privileged women. Indeed, to the extent that those with more resources have greater capacities to care—now by importing it—and so to produce and sustain more capable citizens, the outflow of caregivers may gen-erate profound additional global inequalities in social and politi-cal capacity. As global capital uses particular places for particular forms of reproduction and care workers are cultivated, extracted, and exported for the global marketplace—their labor revalued, repackaged, and relocated—health care systems suffer, the ill and dependent suffer, and family and community life, even political ca-pacities, face erosion.

Host Countries

In the absence of comprehensive data we can only speculate about the implications for the host, or destination, countries. Host coun-tries (that is, their institutions and their populations) clearly benefit to the extent that they get relief, at least temporarily, from labor shortages. This translates into better population health, including the health of those in need of long-term care, than would be possible if the care gap were to remain unfilled. It may be that on some measure this imported labor is cheaper, in that many care workers, especially the less-educated ones, get less than U.S. citizens would receive in the way of pay and benefits. When workers are trained abroad, host countries may also gain substantial savings from not investing in the education of caregivers or in the health sector and social services sector. Proponents of international recruitment, indeed, maintain that there are considerable domestic training cost savings in filling vacant positions with internationally trained health workers, even after accounting for the costs of recruitment and additional training to meet registration standards. Yet the United States and other countries that turn to women educated and trained in the global South potentially neglect domestic investment in education and training. They risk the erosion of their educational capacities and their own capacities to provide care for their populations over time.

A growing body of evidence points to major losses to businesses under current "care regimes" (Ungerson 2004). We can identify both macroeconomic and microeconomic consequences. The United States, analysts argue, "loses a key engine of economic growth because our outdated workplaces push highly trained workers out of the workforce" (Williams and Boushey 2010, 4). Moreover, MetLife and the National Alliance for Caregiving (2006) estimated the total cost to employers in lost productivity due to full-time employees having caregiving responsibilities (this includes replacement costs, absenteeism, interruptions, and so forth) to be more than $33.5 billion. The heightened anxiety and stress of caregivers, paid and unpaid alike, surely also serves as a burden on their families, and more broadly, on the social fabric.

The Dependent Elderly

What of the group we began with, the dependent elderly in high-income countries? As shown in chapter 2, if they get care, it may well be of questionable quality, despite some extraordinary efforts.

Evidence from at least two different directions points to the effect of the current organization of the health care system on the elderly in need of long-term care. First, data reveal profound consequences of care being fragmented and care workers being poorly trained (and often poorly treated): patients do not get needed services; services are duplicated; treatments conflict; and preventable hospitalizations occur (Parry, Coleman, Smith et al. 2003; Boockvar, Fishman, Kyriacou, et al. 2004; Foust, Naylor, Bolling, et al. 2005; Levenson and Saffel 2007). Studies on the effects on quality of long-term care of nurse and other care worker shortages paint a similar picture (Aiken, Clarke, Stone, et al. 2001; Institute of Medicine 2001a; 2001b; Centers for Medicare and Medicaid Services 2002; Needleman, Buerhaus, Mattke, et al. 2002; Institute of Medicine 2003; Wenger, Solomon, Roth, et al. 2003).

Evidence in the United States on the impact of "consumer directed care" suggests that it has generated outcomes that are not worse and perhaps improved in comparison with more traditional models of service delivery (Doty 2004). At the same time, studies on the outcomes of cash-for-care schemes, overall, show that while they vary (depending upon whether workers are regulated and whether payment to relatives is allowed and other contextual factors such as place), the "marketization of intimacy and the commodification of care" can serve to adversely affect the quality of care and transform social relations (Ungerson 1997, 363; Folbre and Nelson 2000; Ungerson 2004).

Looked at ecologically, it seems the trend is toward the global erosion of long-term care, with the gravest consequences for source countries in the South. As poorer countries lose their care workers to wealthier ones, their capacities for care, long-term and other, become diminished. And yet, as wealthier countries benefit from—and increasingly rely on—the transnational flow, they can hardly boast about the quality of their own long-term care capacities.

Long-term Care and Structural Injustice

An overlapping consensus of moral reasons can be marshaled to argue that the current configuration of long-term care is unethical.

We might say that it is wrong because it threatens the well-being or welfare of persons or because it constrains their agency, and in particular their autonomy. We could also express the wrong in terms of threats to human dignity and the ideal of equal moral worth. On a relational account of harm, it becomes clear that the threat accrues not merely to individuals but "by extension, the equal moral standing of their families and communities" (Miller 2009, 512). We might also understand the wrongs here—particularly if we emphasize the global shortage and maldistribution of care workers—in terms of distributive injustice, a failure to equitably allocate human and other resources (Lethbridge 2004; Loriaux 2006; Mackintosh, Mensah, and Rowson 2006).

Each of these accounts captures important aspects of the harm done by the existing organization of long-term care labor. Having, however, approached the organization of long-term care by thinking ecologically and mapping relations between people, policies, and places, we can generate a better, richer account of the harms done here. Ecological thinking, more specifically, traces the operations of structural injustice.

CHAPTER FOUR

An Ecological Ethic

Ecological thinking allows us to trace the structures and processes that organize long-term care labor and connect people around the world: the elderly and their loved ones (mostly daughters) in the North; the poor women, increasingly from the South, who support them; and people needing care in source countries. By starting from interconnections and surveying interrelated social and geographical landscapes, we can see more precisely how, under the current organization of long-term care labor, these groups are imperiled and how care resources, revalued as exports under contemporary global economic models, are flowing away from countries in the global South toward affluent countries like the United States and their citizens with long-term care needs—who are in many cases far from flourishing; and we can see how ultimately this arrangement stands to benefit international lenders and for-profit health care and recruitment corporations and their shareholders.

Resisting reductive and fragmented analyses of "discrete, disparate beings, events, and items in the world . . . only subsequently to propose connections among them or to insert them into 'contexts' conceived as separately given" (Code 2006, 7), ecological thinking suggests new ideas about responsibility for global health equity. Specifically, it helps to shine light on the precise nature of harms done and their operations, and in turn on the sources and the aims of responsibility. In this chapter I explore how responsibilities—diverse in their nature and extent—to address harms flow from the nature of the relationships that obtain between governments, international lending bodies, the for-profit sector, and the other agents situated in the global structures that organize long-term care work. I argue that the grounding of responsibility can be found not merely in shared humanity, compassion, and participation in the processes that generate injustice but also in our nature as interdependent beings who are, in a profound sense, constitutive of one another. Indeed, the social connections between us—"across distance" as they are often framed—are even tighter than most theorizing about global justice acknowledges.

I also want to suggest that, thinking ecologically, the focus of responsibility shifts from individual agents toward ecological subjects, beings who are situated temporally, spatially, and socially and who need particular kinds of habitats in which to become and endure. The idea I argue for, in essence, is that justice in long-term care—and perhaps, also global health equity more generally—calls for ethical place-making for ecological subjects.

Long-term Care and Structural Injustice

As noted at the end of chapter 3, there is no shortage of ways to describe the wrongs done by the existing organization of long-term care. With the benefit of ecological epistemology we can see more clearly the complexity of the social processes and structures that cause harm in patterned and particularized ways and their operations over time. Structural injustice "exists when social processes put large categories of persons under a systematic threat of domination or deprivation of the means to develop and exercise their capacities, at the same time as these processes enable others to dominate or have a wider range of opportunities for developing and exercising their capacities." The ethical concern is not merely that structures constrain; "rather the injustice consists in the *way* they constrain and enable, and how they expand or contract . . . opportunities" (Young 2006, 114).

Social structures serve "as background conditions for individual actions inasmuch as they present actors with options; they provide 'channels' that both enable and constrain. These constraints and enablements occur not only by means of institutional rules and norms enforced by sanctions but also by incentive structures that make some courses of action particularly attractive . . . or make other courses of action particularly costly" (Young 2004b, 9). The people described here, especially those in source countries whose health care systems are failing, are harmed not merely because resources are inequitably distributed or because their self-determination is constrained, or because their equal moral worth is denied or, more broadly, because their welfare interests are threatened. More precisely, they are harmed by the ways in which they are situated amid social norms and economic structures, institutional rules, incentive structures, and sanctions, decision-making processes and routines of interaction, and by the ways these serve systematically to expand opportunities for some while contracting them for others (Young 2006, 114).

There are surely differences in how people experience injustice as individuals, yet the injustice they suffer is both positional and general. Many people are situated in a generalized social position, for example, of being aged and dependent; or not having adequate leave time from an employer to care for family members; or they may be unable to support a family by working in their home country, or may be educated yet have to work below their education level because of the contours of the global labor market; people may have resources to care for loved ones or not have such resources; they may have access to health care and long-term care services or not have such access. Thus, while people make choices, like how and where to work, they are structurally positioned and, accordingly, constrained. It is not the structural positioning that is the problem but rather the systematic contraction of opportunity for some as the opportunities of others expand.

Additionally, there are asymmetries between people in their experience of structural injustice. The dependent elderly in the United States, for instance, are vulnerable, yet less so than those in source countries that have care worker shortages. Family caregivers in the North struggle, to varying degrees, depending, for instance, upon their social and economic status. But they are better situated than emigrant care workers. Workers who are more skilled are better off than the less-skilled; the authorized are better situated than the unauthorized; and so on.

Understanding injustice as structural enables us to trace our relationships and the nature of our relationships to others even across what might seem, from a particular (myopic? nationalistic?) perspective, a great distance. Iris Marion Young's discussion of the relationships that constitute the apparel industry is instructive:

> A complex chain of production and distribution involving dozens of contractually distinct entities bring[s] the clothes manufactured in one place to the stores in which people buy them. . . . The firms higher up the chain . . . often have no legal responsibility for the policies and operations of the firms below with which they contract . . . the workers who make garments are at the bottom of the chain . . . [and] suffer injustice in the form of domination, coercion, and need-deprivation within a global system of vast inequalities. Because of the complexity of the system that brings items from production to sale, and the manner in which the system constrains the options of many of the actors within it, this is an example of *structural* injustice. (2006, 110–11)

The complexity of the processes and relations involved in structural injustice presents challenges when it comes to the work of attributing and assigning responsibilities. Given the way that structures operate, responsibility is diffused or dispersed. It can therefore be difficult if not impossible to identify a particular perpetrator (individual or corporate) to whom particular harms might be traced directly. As Young explains, while "structural processes that produce injustice result from the actions of many persons and the policies of many organizations, in most cases it is not possible to trace which specific actions of which specific agents cause which specific parts of the structural processes or their outcomes" (Young 2006, 115). At the same time, adverse effects are not necessarily intended. Indeed, structural injustice often occurs as a result of our (individual and institutional) choices and actions as we try to advance our own interests "within given institutional rules and accepted norms" (114).[1] To the extent that these effects are foreseeable, however, responsibilities are more easily imposed.

Another challenge of grounding responsibility for structural injustice comes from a specific phenomenology of agency that informs our prevailing conception of responsibility. This phenomenology emphasizes, or "gives experiential primacy" to, effects that emerge in the short-term rather than to remote effects or those that evolve. This is important ethically because when consequences or outcomes are generated by an (often wide) array of agents and unfold over time, our sense of agency diminishes; that is, we see ourselves as implicated very little, if at all (Young 2004a, 373–74).

Transnational Ties, Transnational Responsibilities

The pattern of framing conversations about long-term care policy in nationalist terms ignores the growing reliance on care labor from abroad and its implications, including those for emigrant care workers and, most troublingly, source countries' care systems, institutional and familial. To respond to those who argue that principles of justice cannot apply globally, we can point to dense relations of interdependence that connect people transnationally. There are several ways to think about these relations.

According to Onora O'Neill (2000), an agent's moral obligation encompasses all those people whom his or her particular activities assume—that is, depend upon—and so is often global in scope. According to Thomas Pogge, by "shaping and enforcing the social conditions that foreseeably and avoidably cause the monumental suffering of global poverty, we are harming the global poor" (2005, 33). On this view, our connection is a matter of being "materially involved" in or "substantially contributing to" upholding the institutions responsible for injustice (2004, 137). Young proposes a "social connection model of responsibility" in which "obligations of justice arise between [agents] by virtue of the social processes that connect them" (2006, 102). "All agents," in other words, "who contribute by their actions to the structural processes that produce injustice have responsibilities to work to remedy these injustices" (103).

Consider two examples that draw on the discussion in chapter 3. The first concerns the roles of privileged families in the United States; the second considers histories of colonialism on the current emigration of long-term care workers and the consequent deepening of global health inequities, and perhaps other inequities, too.

Joan Tronto has argued that the tendency among middle-class and more affluent families in the United States to understand caring in private terms—that is, as a matter involving the needs of their loved ones exclusively—can lead to moral hazards, including social harm. "In a competitive society," she observes, "what it means to care well for one's own [family] is to make sure that they have a competitive edge against other [families]" (2006, 10).[2] More privileged people may not be concerned if the caring needs of those who provide them with services go unmet. Ultimately, those acting with what Tronto describes as "privileged irresponsibility" "ignore the ways in which their own caring activities continue to perpetuate inequality" (13). It seems fair to assume that affluent family caregivers in the United States are not trying to cause global suffering; they are only trying to do the best for their loved ones. In a context of structural injustice, however, they participate in perpetuating it. As we have seen, though, they do so to a great extent because they are constrained by workplace practices.

Turning to the second example, postcolonial theorists maintain that conversations on the topic of care worker emigration tend to obscure the extent to which this "draws upon colonial legacies to make up the postcolonial present," which serves to "disavow . . . the interdependent relationships . . . established over centuries of co-production of medical care across different parts of the Empire" (Raghuram 2009, 30), relationships that expand possibilities for some while contracting them for others.

We might also consider relationships of responsibility between international financial institutions whose "development" projects claim to generate benefits for source countries, including their health care systems; or between U.S.-based health and long-term care corporations who recruit abroad and patients in source countries; or perhaps between businesses in the United States with family caregivers in their ranks and the well-being of their loved ones; or between these businesses and patients in source countries serving the United States. Ties are indirect. Harms tend not to be intentional, direct, or swiftly identifiable. Responsibilities are hard, then, to trace. Ecological thinking gives us the needed resources.

Global Equality of What?

So far I have argued that we need to understand injustice in long-term care as structural and responsibility as global. What, then, should we aim for in addressing injustice—that is, global injustice in long-term care and, perhaps, by extension, global health equity? Contemporary work on justice has shifted away from thinking strictly about the distribution of resources, or what people have, toward their capacities, or what they "are able to do and to be" (Nussbaum 2006, 70). What I will call "enabling" conceptions of justice aim at attending to the social and political conditions that support people's capacities for self-development and self-determination. Young's theory of justice as enablement calls for reform of the social and institutional structures that systematically constrain people's capacities for self-development and self-determination. Carol Gould's notion of justice as "equal positive freedom" requires not only "the absence of constraining conditions such as coercion and oppression" but also access to the means or conditions for "self-transformation" and the "development of capacities and the realization of projects over time." Justice, here too, is about "the availability of *enabling* [my emphasis] conditions" for individuals (Gould 2009, 165–66). Finally, Nussbaum and Sen's capabilities approach (2006), a minimalist, agent-centered, universalistic account of global justice, emphasizes people's capacities to be and to do. As Nussbaum underscores, here "active striving" and "achievement" matter (73).

Jennifer Ruger's work on global health inequalities has also embraced this emphasis on supporting individuals' "beings and doings" through a concept of health capabilities (Ruger 2006). Global health inequalities are morally troubling, here, because deprivations in the capability to function threaten individuals' well-being, defined as having capabilities to achieve a range of beings and doings, or the freedom to be what the individual wants to be and do what he or she wants to do (999). Justice requires that a society provides people "with the necessary conditions for achieving the highest possible threshold level of health so they can have flourishing lives" (1002).

In a related vein, in proposing a moral framework to guide future progress toward the Millenium Development Goals, for example, Jeffrey Waage and his colleagues argue for a view of "development" "as a dynamic process involving sustainable and equitable access to improved well-being . . . that is, the freedom to enjoy various combinations of beings and doings . . . [or] to make choices and act effectively" (Waage, Banjeri, and Campbell 2010, 1009).

I want to suggest that discussions of the aims of enabling conceptions of justice suffer from an impoverished conception of the targets of the work of justice, and do so because they fail to reckon fully with interdependence, locatedness (structural and spatial), and temporality. We need an ecological understanding of subjects.

Ecological Subjects and Ethical Place-making

As Code explains it, the ecological subject is an embodied, temporal subject who is socially and spatially situated, for whom "locatedness and interdependence are integral to its possibilities." Ecological subjects, indeed, are "made by and mak[e our] relations in reciprocity with other subjects *and* [my emphasis] with . . . (multiple, diverse) locations" (Code 2006, 128). These processes of forging are shaped by the realities of our embeddedness within a particular social and material environment and the forces of temporality; they are, at the same time, matters of some choice.

An ecological conception of the subject, then, first should replace the conception of the person found in much liberal moral and political philosophy that emphasizes rationality, independence or self-reliance, and that assumes equality among us. This idealization renders the body irrelevant and tends to ignore our inherently social nature, including the necessity of relations of dependence. Furthermore, it obscures the profound relations of inequality that abound. People are far from being similarly situated, as we have seen. Nussbaum, Young, and, I take it, Ruger, are not guilty of these forms of myopia, but their emphasis on the self in articulating the ideals of global justice still serves to obscure our interdependence and need for caring relations.[3] In a global economic order marked by the retraction of the public sector and a growing emphasis on individual responsibility for self-care, upholding self-development and self-determination as ideals, should, indeed, give us pause. Too, their emphasis on individual choice and activity, including "striving," "achievement," and "transformation," may eclipse other possibilities for the substance of a good life.

Even though references to activities such as "development" and "striving" suggest some acknowledgment of our temporality, the emphasis on "being" (well-being) might also serve to obscure the fact that we, our interactions, and the social, economic, and political processes in which we are embedded have a past and are ongoing, opening into the future under ever-changing conditions.

We need a conception of the person that highlights the significance of the body, our social nature, and temporality and points to "a fundamental role of all societies [viz.], to provide the circumstances under which humans can be cared for and thrive, given their differing degrees of frailty and vulnerability" over time and through change (Kittay 2002, 78). Less-idealized conceptions, like the notion of the ecological subject, will allow us to formulate ideals for global justice with more traction.

If we jettison the excessive emphasis on "self," "being," and notions of achievement and mastery and shift our attention to the idea that we are interdependent subjects with a temporal, creative, generative nature, we might describe justice as enablement through the concepts of "becoming" and "enduring" (Bergson 1911); that is, our capacities for becoming and enduring in cohabitation with others. Becoming can be understood as having the capacity for processes of development, evolution, and expansion (Grosz 1999). Duration encompasses capacities for sustaining ongoing processes of "conservation, resilience, preservation, and abiding" (Casey 1999, 218).[4] Decision, action, and mastery are not necessarily—though they could be—what gives life meaning and value for ecological subjects. The concepts of becoming and duration leave open more possibilities. Both unfold over time. Each of them can occur only in concert with other ecological subjects. Moreover, each can be precarious, or perhaps impossible, depending upon how subjects are situated in social structures and in particular geographic locations, or "habitats."[5]

Indeed, bodies and caring relations are not the whole story for ecological subjects. *Places* have to meet certain conditions if ecological subjects are to survive, not to mention realize justice.[6] Rosemarie Garland-Thomson's notion of the "misfit" helps to shed light on the idea. Our shared vulnerability is not, she argues, just in our embodiment and potential to suffer, but in the need for "fit" between our bodies and our environments. "Misfits" are those who are ensconced in environments that cannot sustain them, or when, as she puts it, "the world fails the flesh" (Garland-Thomson 2010).

Ecological subjects cannot survive or thrive in the absence of functioning, effective public health and health care systems and care relations, and they may struggle to do so when environments—social, institutional, and other—are impoverished, constituted to narrowly define their possibilities and/or constrain their abilities to meet their needs and the needs of their loved ones. Thinking ecologically therefore reveals the need to resist an excessive emphasis on individuals as the primary focus of efforts aimed at justice. Such efforts cannot be lucidly conceived apart from our relationality and embeddedness in movement through social (transnational) processes and places. I expand on this point below.

Thinking ecologically also reveals the need to take seriously the "rhizomatic structure of [our] implacement" (Casey 1997, 337); that is, the reality that we live within and continually navigate a set of relations between places: homes, places of work, care settings, borders, and so on. Ecological subjects can suffer from social structures and processes that create fragmentation or cause rupture.

A third dimension of ecological subjectivity involves what geographers have called the "intersubjectivity" of place. Seeing place in relational terms—that is, as intersubjectively constructed—"highlights the multiplicity of locations as well as the variety of interactions between people who are located differently that go into making places" (Raghuram, Madge, and Noxolo 2009, 8). This is significant ethically because it raises questions about *responsibilities* "for those relations with other parts of the world through which . . . identit[ies] are formed" (Massey 2004, 13). As Massey argues, to the extent that we are "constitutively, elements within a wider, configurational, distributed geography . . . that raises a second question [concerning] . . . the geography of relations through which any particular identity is established and maintained" (2006, 93).

Just as the development of "global cities" has spawned "survival circuits" (Sassen 2002a) and drained poor parts of the globe of their populations to serve the privileged classes under global economic structures, the burgeoning need for health care workers in the United States and elsewhere in the affluent world is threatening the availability of care in low- and some middle-income countries, shaping and potentially eroding parts of the social and institutional landscape in particular ways in particular countries. While most accounts point to our shared humanity or our participation in processes that generate injustice, ecological thinking offers a more robust way of understanding our connections under globalization and thus provides new resources for grounding responsibilities for global justice. We are responsible for global health equity perhaps not (merely) because of our humanity and/or participation in processes that generate injustice but also because of who and what we are as ecological subjects: creatures whose identities and habitats are not merely relational but intersubjectively constructed; indeed, mutually constitutive.

In light of these considerations, I suggest that responsibility for justice in long-term care—and even global health at large—might best be conceived as involving "ethical place-making" (Massey 2006; Raghuram, Madge, Noxolo 2009, 7) for ecological subjects. Thoroughly fleshing out the meaning of this phrase—coined by geographers—and its significance for global health equity warrants a separate project. Here, I offer a mere sketch.

Place, at least on philosophical accounts, "is no fixed thing" (Casey 1997, 286). It can be understood as being *around* us, as the commonsense view has it, but also *in* and *with* us. That is to say, *place* may refer to geographic regions and built places such as institutional care settings and workplaces. Jacques Derrida, writing on architecture, speaks of "scenographies of passage" where "passage connotes movement between places [and] . . . a place *through which* to pass" (Casey 1997, 313). We might also draw insight from the notion, developed by Gilles Deleuze and Felix Guattari, of "nomad space" to capture the experience of those who are in some sense distributed between places, who are at once "here/there *and* there/here" (ibid. 305), yet who, as noted earlier, may see themselves as having "a foot here, a foot there, a foot *nowhere* [my emphasis]" (DiCicco-Bloom 2004, 28).

An account of justice for long-term care, and perhaps global health generally, that reckons with our "implacement" calls for situating ecological subjects (here, family caregivers, their loved ones in need of assistance, and care workers) within and between particular-yet-interconnected places: homes, places of work, institutional care settings, recruiting offices, immigration facilities, and so on, in both source and destination countries and making more equal the conditions that support becoming and duration. This means, more specifically, refraining from creating conditions of deprivation (that is conditions that cannot support and sustain capacities for becoming and enduring); supporting conditions that facilitate and sustain becoming and duration; and promoting conditions for ending deprivation and facilitating and sustaining becoming and duration. Justice, it must be underscored, cannot be realized merely by refraining from interference or avoiding the imposition of "systems" or "orders" that prevent others from achieving opportunities. It requires active intervention. If we embrace such an alternative moral ontology and think of ourselves less as independent, self-contained individuals or loosely connected ones or, worse, polarized ones and instead start from notions of embodied subjects situated in interdependent habitats and networks of responsibility and care (Robinson 2006; Sevenhuijsen, Bozalek, Gouws, et al. 2006), the potential for global justice in long-term care seems far more ripe.

The Benefits of an Ecological Ethic

The ecological subject is only "a distant relative" of the disembodied, unlocated and unlocateable, "interchangeable" subject that appears in liberal moral and political theory (Code 2006, 5) and that haunts many policy discussions. By reckoning with our embodied and sociospatially situated nature, this account resists tendencies to privilege particular, culturally dominant conceptions of persons and their most vital capacities and instead allows for paying careful attention to particularities of people and places. It allows for contextually sensitive explorations of how it is and should be for ecological subjects in the many places they inhabit and traverse, striving to become and endure. Because for ecological subjects, meanings and expressions of becoming and enduring, of harm, and so forth are "situated" socially and constituted relationally (Miller 2009), robust, egalitarian decision-making processes and responsive institutions and interactions are necessary to determine what precisely is needed in particular places for particular people; that is, justice demands fair processes for asking: What would ethical place-making mean here, or here, or here?

With the capacities to "become" and "endure" as universal norms and egalitarian processes for deciding on their precise content, indeed, we can avoid ageism and a kind of neocolonialism offered with a caring face. When it comes to the dependent elderly, self-determination and self-transformation may be dangerous ideals at which to aim in long-term care policy, given social norms—and to some extent physical realities—that see the elderly as being in a state of ultimate cognitive and physical decline. Especially in an environment of cost-cutting, such ideals also may well leave them vulnerable to some notion that they can be left to fend for themselves. In a culture already marked by an emphasis on self-reliance, this seems especially likely (von Mering 1996). The discourse of self-development and self-determination has been used to shape migrant care workers and source countries into the kinds of "empowered" economic agents sought after by the architects of the global economy (Schild 2007). When countries are described as "developing," the implication is that they are behind and working to "catch up." This framing suggests that people globally are in some sort of queue, obscuring the relations of inequality that generate and perpetuate deprivation and suppress ideas about alternative futures (Massey 2006). Under the banner of self-development and self-determination, global economic structures have already imperiled, and stand to do so further, the dependent elderly, family caregivers, emigrant care workers, and their home countries through the "shifting of responsibility for social risks onto [them as] individuals, and transforming [what had been understood as social] responsibility into a problem of self-care" (Schild 2007, 199).

Moreover, to the extent that received accounts of global justice, including arguments focused on global health equity, use *well-being* and *flourishing* interchangeably, the proposal here seems appropriately ambitious in not aiming at the higher ideal of flourishing but taking seriously prospects greater than mere subsistence. Identifying norms that can be discussed and institutionalized sooner rather than later seems crucial, given the severity of the injustice some people face under contemporary conditions (Parekh 2008, 107).

Maybe most important, the recognition in this account of the intersubjectivity of place offers new resources for grounding responsibilities for global justice. While most accounts point to our shared humanity, feelings of compassion or benevolence for others (Nussbaum 2006; Gould 2007a; 2007b), or our participation in processes that generate injustice (Pogge 2004; Young 2006), ecological thinking offers a more robust way of understanding our connections under globalization. We should accept responsibilities for justice and for global health equity not merely because of our shared humanity, our feelings for others, or our contribution to injustice, but also because of who and what we are as ecological subjects: creatures whose identities and dwelling places are not merely relational but intersubjectively constructed, indeed, mutually constitutive.

What we find, then, by thinking ecologically, is that even where the governments and citizenry of wealthy countries, along with other agents whose policies and practices have global reach, are not motivated by moral arguments, they may be moved by *prudential* arguments that acknowledge our interdependence. Indeed, these agents have prudential reasons to care about the health status of care workers, their access to good education and training, their treatment by labor and immigration policies, even if only for the sake of the quality of care for the aged and dependent in destination countries. And because not all care workers trained abroad emigrate, the local populations in source countries potentially can benefit if the health care infrastructure in these countries meets high standards for education and training. I hasten to add that prudential arguments will likely not be able to address all the concerns raised here. Yet they can surely serve the purpose of motivating at least some action toward justice. Although I would prefer that things be otherwise, given urgent realities on the ground, especially in low-income source countries, I am prepared to put forward this minimalist view in the hope that it will foster appreciation for our profound interdependence.[7]

Yet another benefit of thinking ecologically is that, by being able to trace more precisely the connections between those who contribute to and suffer from injustice, we are in a better position to assign responsibilities whose nature and extent vary. "Differences in kind and degree" of responsibilities "correlate with an agent's position within the structural processes" (Young 2006, 126); and, we can add, the geography of long-term care and care worker emigration. The questions for justice concern how we are connected and what are our capacities. I elaborate on this in the next chapter.

Along with putting us in a better position to acknowledge and attend to interdependencies and particularities among people and places with an ecological conception of subjects, an ecological notion of citizenship might enable some forms of political recognition more appropriate to a globalizing world. We can accommodate the millions of migrant care workers who, whatever their origins, contribute significantly to the sustenance of more than one habitat and who may think of themselves as hybrids or as having a cosmopolitan identity (Young 2000, 236–37).

Finally, an approach to global or cosmopolitan justice for long-term care that focuses on sustaining places that support capacities for becoming and enduring strikes the right balance between acknowledging the past and privileging the future. In its very structure, it aims at ensuring a future; indeed, a more equitable one. This would represent a major advance in global public health policy and planning. As critics have observed generally (Graham 2010), and with respect to long-term care specifically (WHO 2002a; 2002c; Miller, Booth, and Mor 2008), the future is strikingly absent from view. At the same time, on this view we see more clearly the relationship between the past, present, and future and so can hold those who have contributed to injustice accountable for past wrongs so they can contribute to justice in the future. The moral attitude is not so much one of blame, which could undermine efforts to address injustice through its more adversarial posture (Young 2006), but rather acknowledgment and (inevitably situated) engaged reflection on our ongoing connections. It invites us to ask not just "what has been done?" but also "what has not been done?" (Young 2004a, 376). In my final chapter, I outline some possibilities.

CHAPTER FIVE

Realizing Justice Globally in Long-term Care

How can we move forward, having shifted the lens so that the focus is a bit less on individual agents and a bit more on their interdependence with others and need for certain kinds of habitats, places in which they can become and endure under conditions of equality? Who are the responsible agents and what are they to do?

I have argued that an ecological approach reveals the injustice of current arrangements in long-term care—injustice that is structural in form, and experienced by the elderly, family members who co-ordinate and provide care, and members of the paid long-term care workforce, especially emigrants, as well as populations in source countries. The ecological approach suggests a way forward, toward establishing a new ethical norm for future policy and planning in long-term care and perhaps, too, efforts aimed at global health equity generally. Responsibility, on the view I have proposed, should be conceived as ethical place-making for ecological subjects; that is, making more equal the conditions for the becoming and duration of interdependent people in particular places.

Assigning Responsibilities for Shared Health Governance

Typically, in discussions of global justice, including discussions of global health equity, states are assumed to have primary responsibility; that is, the "most direct and prior obligations" (Ruger 2006, 1001). Yet states' limitations are many: some states do not have the capability to ensure justice, some lack the desire, and some states with the desire to be just are rendered more porous by neoliberal policies and programs and, so, are constrained in their capacities by the activities of other agents operating within them (O'Neill 2004, 246–47). Some argue that international lending bodies and transnational corporations now may have an even greater influence on health than governments and the World Health Organization (People's Health Movement 2005). Transnational corporations, nongovernmental organizations, international lending bodies, and other global actors and institutions should therefore serve along with states as primary agents of justice.

Indeed, all "*dwelling* [my emphasis] in this institutional and causal nexus," and who thus constitute and are constituted by the people and places suffering injustice, are responsible (Young 2000, 224). This includes governments and global institutions, along with nongovernmental organizations, businesses, and foundations, as well as families and individuals. Addressing injustice in long-term care and global health requires collective action, or what we should call "shared health governance" (Ruger 2006, 1001), aimed at cultivating more equal conditions for those who need and those who provide long-term and other care to become and endure as they navigate and dwell in such places as homes, workplaces, long-term care institutions, and other care settings, within particular regions, communities, and the places between them, including, for some, immigration offices and borders.

An agent's position within the structural process and in the geography of long-term care help to determine the nature and extent of responsibilities. The social connection model of responsibility enriched with ecological thinking's demand for attention to the relational nature of identities and place offers a method: agents should examine their particular structural as well as geographical positioning and how they are situated in relation to those suffering injustice to determine their responsibilities and range of opportunities for contribution based on their scope of power, resources, and privilege.[1]

Agents like international bodies, states, domestic institutions, for-profit agents, and other collectivities can at most focus on the "positional and general" justice that people suffer and target those structural and geographic locations. We should think in terms of the responsibilities of U.S. employers to their employees; of U.S. policymakers to employers and employees and to the aging; and of U.S. health care corporations and institutions, the U.S. government, the World Bank and International Monetary Fund (IMF), source country governments (where functioning effectively), and for-profit recruiters, individually and collectively, to potential recruits and to the poor needing long-term and other varieties of care in source countries. In our personal interactions—for example, between high-income family members and the particular care workers supporting their loved ones; between particular employers and employees; and between individual recruiters and would-be migrant nurses—we can offer more finely tuned interventions aimed at justice. I elaborate on this below.

It fits with our moral intuitions to hold that those who not only contribute to but benefit significantly from injustice have special responsibilities. Those responsible in this manner include governments who save on health and care workforce investment, the beneficiaries of international lending bodies' practices, unscrupulous employers and recruiters who profit from the migration of poor workers, and affluent families in the United States. All of these are more able than others by virtue of their structural positioning and consequent greater privilege "to adapt to changed circumstances without suffering serious deprivation" (Young 2006, 128).

International lending bodies, principally the World Bank and the

IMF, should reconsider practices of placing constraining conditions on loans and rescind the requirement on debtor countries to cut public spending on things like food for the poor and education. They should also contribute to rebuilding public health systems with more egalitarian and responsive institutions designed to determine local needs, including needs for long-term care.

The global health system ("the constellation of actors [individuals and/or organizations] whose primary purpose is to promote, restore or maintain health" [WHO 2006a]) should gather and disseminate data on care work and its impact socially, economically, and politically and help to show the ways in which care work, including long-term care, is a core public need and not merely a private concern as constructed under neoliberalism. They should gather and disseminate information on models for incorporating and integrating care in the social and economic infrastructure of particular countries as well as highlight relationships—interdependencies and patterns—between and among countries and regions. They should convene agents and facilitate conversations around care planning, including workforce and other resource needs, and determine the needs of the care workforce globally, regionally, and locally, encouraging attention to patterns and particularities among people and places; establish and promulgate standards for health workforce planning and education, worker recruitment and emigration, and working conditions for care workers. They should also exert pressure on international lenders and transnational corporations to eliminate injustice-generating policies and practices.

Given the shifting landscape of global health, the World Health Organization (WHO) is exploring new models for collaborating with its member states, other international bodies and organizations, civil society, and the private sector. To date, the WHO has issued reports on models of care and the role of informal care (Wiener 2003). Along with the Milbank Memorial Fund, the WHO has recently launched an International Long-term Care Initiative (2009) that aims to establish broad principles for long-term care. It does not address the issues raised by unprecedented migration, however. The organization has also issued a draft Code of Practice on the International Recruitment of Health Personnel (2008; Eckenwiler 2009). Concern over the aging of the Caribbean population inspired the Pan American Health Organization and the Merck Institute of Aging and Health to formulate a plan to improve monitoring the health of the elderly, develop a public health research agenda to identify threats to the health of the elderly, establish a regulatory framework for protecting them in long-term care settings, and improve health workforce training around their needs (Pan American Health Organization 2004c). These important initiatives may well generate significant improvements in long-term care. Yet they are still largely isolated and narrowly targeted efforts that fail to challenge the global economic and immigration policies largely responsible for the injustice facing family caregivers, paid care workers, and source countries.

Joining and in some cases challenging the efforts of the usual suspects in the global health arena like the WHO and PAHO is a growing mix of civil society and nongovernmental organizations, private firms, and private philanthropists (Szlezák, Bloom, Jamison, et al. 2010). For example, the Development Action for Women Network (DAWN) provides assistance to women migrants—primarily Filippinas—and promotes their "issues, rights, and concerns" (2010). DAWN offers advocacy and information, counseling, educational, financial, and legal assistance, and a range of trainings, seminars, and workshops aimed at promoting justice for women migrants.

Labor organizations and trade unions like the International Labour Organization (ILO) and Service Employees International Union (SEIU) should persist in their efforts to organize workers and secure better workplace conditions for care workers and for family members with responsibilities for care.

New global institutions might be developed. The "global household," defined as "an institution formed by family networks dispersed across national boundaries [and] composed of nuclear and extended families and friends," is one possibility (Safri and Graham 2010, 100). Given its role in generating substantial social and economic wealth in the form of care and other unpaid household labor (often coordinated and provided transnationally) and remittances, the global household clearly "participates in international production, finance, and trade in addition to the coordination of international migration" (ibid.). What if we were to regard the global household as an agent with status equal to a multinational firm? What if, along with the International Labour Organization, for instance, there was a Global Household Organization? Such an organization could raise for discussion issues around migration, household maintenance, the division of labor, decision-making authority over the use of resources, the impact of remittances, members' needs for care, the interactions between households and other global agents, and so forth (119–20). Safri and Graham argue that treating the global household as an actor in the global economy "strengthens the vision of globalization from below; alters the participants, practices, and potentials of economic development; and reconfigures the imaginary of economic transformation" (100). Similarly, the vast numbers of women who make up much of the global health workforce, if organized, would likely be a potent global economic and political force.

The United States and other countries must participate in efforts at the global level to manage their long-term care needs and promote health equity. The United States, in particular, should exert influence with the World Bank, the World Trade Organization, and the WHO to advance reform. There are already established commitments, in the form of international health agreements, and even emergent government-sponsored initiatives aimed at global health that can serve as the basis for action. The United States is a signatory to the Millennium Development Goals (MDGs), the Group of Eight Health Commitments, and has expressed support at least for the International Health Partnership, tied to the promotion of the MDGs (Kaiser Family Foundation 2010b). The U.S. Global Health Initiative, launched in 2010, lists a women- and girl-centered approach at the top of its list of core principles (Kaiser Family Foundation 2010a). Other principles emphasize integration and coordination and sustainability, following a call to "take advantage of synergies" (3). Although it adopts a disease-based approach to identifying target areas, it does include among them health-system strengthening. Each of these existing commitments can and should serve as grounds for action on the issues raised here.

Beyond participating in global dialogue and coordinated action with other institutional agents on global health, governments are responsible for making a central place for humans' shared need for care in environs that support capacities for becoming and duration for all their citizens and residents. Embracing an ecological approach to policy making, they should engage in more careful long-term planning for the long-term care workforce and incorporate and integrate concern for care across policy sectors, especially those of health, economics, labor, and immigration. Ecological thinking at the government level might also serve to promote strategies that integrate decision making and care for the dependent elderly and that strive to ensure that the places they inhabit can sustain them and support their ongoing efforts to become, even near the end of life. It could facilitate the development of strategies to support employers, who could, in turn, better support their employees who have caregiving responsibilities. It could help to avoid stopgap measures that perpetrate and perpetuate injustice abroad, such as turning to low-income countries to meet workforce needs (see, for example, Yan 2006; Academy Health 2008). And for foreign-educated care workers who emigrate, thinking ecologically could generate policy reforms that ensure essential protections and promote their equality. Most broadly, and also importantly, it could transform what is now essentially a private issue for individuals and families into a matter of central public concern.

Thoughtful recommendations for more comprehensive and coordinated long-term care policy at the country level abound (Levine 1999; Asch, Blustein, and Wasserman 2008; Institute of Medicine 2008; Miller, Brown, and Mor 2008). These include recommendations concerning the integration of long-term care services with other health and social services, better compensation and working conditions for direct care workers, and coalition-building (Kane 2003; Folbre 2006; IOM 2008). A call for nurses to be more capable leaders in long-term care settings and to serve as "connectors" or "integrators" "across the silos of care that exist . . . and enhancing the capacity of the *overall system* to manage complex health conditions *across settings and over time* [my emphases]" (Harvath, Swafford, Smith, et al. 2008; Reinhard and Young 2009, 165) is an encouraging development. Government action is the best-suited to promote such initiatives.

The U.S. Patient Protection and Affordable Care Act of 2010 (PPACA) includes important elements that aim at supporting continuity of care and better quality care for the elderly (SCAN Foundation 2010). This law incorporates measures for improving the coordination of those eligible for both Medicare and Medicaid, for instance. The CLASS plan (Community Living Assistance Services and Supports) allows for the purchase of community living assistance services and supportive resources. Provisions in the PPACA also allocate funding to expand states' aging and disability resource centers, create incentives for states to offer more home and community-based care as an alternative to nursing homes, and invest in the health care workforce. Currently though, initiatives, even ones that provide greater integration, continue to be isolated, giving scant attention to the relationship between the role of families, the workplace, immigration issues, and the interdependence with, and impact on, source countries.

In the realm of family caregiver policy, efforts are dispersed. Organizations like the Family Caregiver Alliance have issued sound policy statements aimed at government officials, albeit framed in nationalist terms (n.d.b). The Centers for Medicare and Medicaid and the Veterans Administration have developed caregiving initiative; the National Family Caregiver Support Program (NFCSP) has been expanded for veterans' families in the wake of the wars in Iraq and Afghanistan; ideas for retirement-savings reform have been floated. Still, as the Institute of Medicine has argued, "while a number of programs and policies either directly or indirectly influence the well-being of informal caregivers, the support programs that exist are generally small, poorly-funded, and fragmented across the federal, state, and local levels" (2008, 260) (Feinberg and Newman 2006).

Justice calls for integrated federal health, economic, and labor policy that supports caregivers and ensures that caring for a loved one will not over time impoverish them, make them anxious and ill, distort their relationships by commodifying them, or thwart their aspirations. This means support for their relations with paid care-givers, restructuring of the health care system to meet long-term care needs, and savings vehicles—payment vehicles that do not dis-tort relationships and that provide meaningful financial support. With an ecological conception, attention to differences among fam-ily caregivers and their particular environs is crucial.

At or near the top of the list should be reform of policies around family leave. Employers should be supported by government in ef-forts to craft workplace conditions that demonstrate respect for the work of care, develop strategies where possible that allow employ-ees flexibility, and offer more robust policies related to family leave. Policies that would allow family caregivers both short-term and ex-tended leaves, including paid leave, more flexibility when they are working, and prohibit discrimination against them are warranted (Rosenfeld 2007; Williams and Boushey 2010). This would pro-mote justice for family caregivers and could also serve to reduce the need for paid care workers from countries who can ill afford to have them leave. Expanding such policies to cover more employ-ees and exploring ways to strengthen such benefits are essential to making leave more accessible and effective.

Policies like this not only promote justice; they also improve workplace productivity. Indeed, figures released by the Confedera-tion of British Industry (CBI) show real benefits to businesses. The CBI Employment Trends Survey of 2008 found that businesses that allowed employees to request flexible working conditions so they could provide care for loved ones found that 69 percent reported a positive impact on employee relations; 63 percent reported a positive impact on recruitment and retention; 35 percent reported a positive impact on absence rates; and 28 percent reported a positive impact on productivity. British Telecom, an industry leader in supporting family caregivers, found a savings of GBP6,000 (approx. $10,000) for each employee who worked at home, increases in productivity of more than 20 percent from these workers, and turnover that was four times lower than the average (Carers UK 2009). One chief executive argued: "By working smarter, and offering real opportunities for people to transform the way they work, employers can reduce costs, as well as help retain their most skilled staff at a time when [given that many family caregivers are at their greatest level of skill and experience] they can least afford to lose them" (Carers UK and Centre for Social Inclusion 2006; Carers UK 2009).

Policymakers and planners might also give more attention to the built environment and work to address the difficulty many family caregivers face in traversing urban, suburban, and rural landscapes to visit their loved ones when they live in the same community. This may sound idealistic. Yet when we consider the impact on family caregivers and the elderly of current configurations, along with the environmental implications of our current patterns of mobility, it becomes ethically necessary.

Justice also calls for government policies that require equal pay, benefits, and worker protection for emigrant care workers with training and responsibilities equivalent to those who are native (Iredale 2005). It calls further for reform of immigration policy that denies them political rights and undermines access to citizenship given their contribution to the very foundation of social organization and cooperation (Tronto 2006; Patterson 2009).

Governments, with the aid of global health organizations, should also work to achieve greater justice by exploring ways of regulating the flow of care workers from low- and middle-income countries to wealthy ones.[2] A select few countries, in collaboration with other countries or organizations, have already begun to design interventions. Voluntary codes of practice and position statements aimed at protecting the health systems of source countries from unethical recruiters and employers are a popular approach. Currently nearly 20 documents have been developed by governments (the United Kingdom is one example), associations of governments (such as the Commonwealth countries), nongovernmental organizations (the International Council of Nurses, for instance), and health professional associations (such as the WHO and the American Public Health Association). While such instruments reflect a commitment to address at least some of the problems associated with health worker emigration and can raise the level of discourse, a major limit is that they are voluntary.

Moreover, the structure and financing of a country's health system is a significant factor when it comes to scope. In the United Kingdom, for example, which has one major public-sector employer and one point of entry for health professionals, a code may have more of an impact than in countries with a wide array of independent private-sector health care employers (Buchan, Parkin, and Sochalski 2003). Given the structure of the health system in the United States, voluntary codes are unlikely to be effective. It may be that only the force of law will allow for ethical recruitment and employment practices for care workers from the global South. Legislation would need to be aimed at public and private employers in health care as well as at for-profit recruitment companies.

Perhaps the most important mechanisms embraced by governments are legally binding bilateral or multilateral agreements. These involve agreements for supplies of health professionals from particular countries (specifically, not those with a low population/care worker ratio and/or high disease burdens) for specified lengths of time to address particular skill shortages. The United Kingdom and South Africa, for example, have a bilateral agreement, and some European Union countries have multilateral agreements. The United States, by contrast, has what might be described as a unilateral policy, involving special visa incentives for nurses but generally no organized strategy on managing international care worker recruitment. There is emerging evidence that shifts in state policy can have significant effects on labor strategies and immigration trends (Bach 2010).

A suggested but still untried strategy involves compensation, wherein governments of host or destination countries would pay source countries for the investments made in educating health professionals (Bundred and Levitt 2000; Stilwell, Diallo, Zurn, et al. 2004). Yet this fails to address the structural factors that generate injustices, and it is not at all clear that it would benefit the health sector specifically.

One other proposal, aimed at the medical "brain drain" in particular, is to organize the curriculum of medical students in low- and middle-income countries around "locally relevant" needs and capacities (Eyal and Hurst 2008). This idea has many virtues, chiefly that it might deepen their appreciation for local needs and engage the schools in efforts to reduce health disparities. At the same time, however, its potential to promote and perhaps perpetuate a kind of institutionalized educational deprivation and disable their efforts to keep up with global advances is worrisome. Although some argue that the education is "inflated" in being oriented around the needs of affluent markets, I maintain that health workers should have the opportunity to receive the best-available education, which includes but is not limited to what is deemed "locally relevant," and that health care resources, including them, should be reallocated more equitably. This provokes crucial questions regarding what kind of a resource a care worker is and should be under globalization—that is, a domestic resource or a global resource—and what implications this has for oversight and investment in health worker education. A global vision with shared governance that attends to particularity is needed here. While self-sufficiency may be unrealistic, source countries should receive from destination countries some clearly defined benefits that they find to be fair.

The long-term care institutions and agencies that employ nurses and direct care workers also must be engaged. They should embrace justice-promoting hiring and workplace practices. They should, in addition, call upon industry groups currently lobbying for the recruitment of care workers from abroad to devote themselves instead to advocating for investment in the domestic care workforce.

Individual citizens of the affluent countries like the United States to which care workers emigrate also have responsibilities to promote justice in this context. As members of a democracy, citizens should call upon elected officials to enact domestic reforms that would ensure living wages and good working conditions for care workers. They should also call for the undocumented to have access to public benefits, including health insurance coverage. Citizens should ask their representatives to address international policies and programs that generate injustice for care workers and those in need of care in the global South, especially programs promulgated by the United States, currently the most powerful member of the IMF and the World Bank. Those who rely on care workers have special responsibilities to advocate for such reforms. Justice also calls for a more equitable distribution of labor within families, so that women do not bear a disproportionate burden of caregiving.

A Place for Practices

We also have responsibilities to avoid perpetuating injustice against, and find ways to promote justice for, care workers in our personal interactions and exchanges with them. Theories of justice that emphasize states and institutions as the primary agents and hold political-legal-institutional reform to be the core work of global justice underestimate the potential of personal interactions and practices among individuals.

Fuyuki Kurasawa critiques a "formalist bias" that involves understanding global justice as emerging principally through prescriptive or legislative means. According to Kurasawa, this overlooks "the social labour and modes of practice that supply the ethical and political soil within which the norms, institutions and procedures of global justice are rooted" (Kurasawa 2007, 6). Modes of practice, he argues, "are the lynchpins of the work of global justice, the points of contact, transmission and mutual influence between national and global institutions . . . at one level, and civil society . . . at the other" (197). These practice modes are best understood as "processes of permanent invention of social relations, searching to generate new structural arrangements and ethical principles as well as different kinds of political action connected to global justice" (199). While governments, international financial institutions, and other corporate agents may have more resources and a greater scope of power, ordinary individuals also have responsibilities from which they "should not be absolved" (Young 2004a, 382). Participation in practices provides one avenue.

A practice, to be more precise, "represents—and simultaneously produces—a pattern of materially and symbolically oriented social action that agents undertake within organized political, cultural and socio-economic fields, and whose main features are recognizable across several temporal and spatial settings. A practice confronts certain perils (or obstacles) and must therefore enact a certain repertoire of social tasks, the whole forming . . . a mode of practice" (Kurasawa 2007, 11–12). Kurasawa identifies several examples: bearing witness, forgiveness, preventive foresight, giving aid, and solidarity. Preventive foresight and solidarity are key practices for promoting justice in long-term care. To these two I will add four more: recognition, appreciation, empathy, and reciprocity.

Justice calls for individuals and families to practice *preventive foresight*. As Kurasawa defines it, this practice is "a sort of farsighted labour constituted through social processes whereby numerous associative groups in national and global civil societies are simultaneously creating and putting into practice a sense of responsibility for the future by attempting to anticipate and avoid severe and structurally based injustices and crises" (2007, 97). Governments, employers, and other collective agents should, for the sake of justice as well as efficiency, embrace it.

Individuals should practice preventive foresight and plan ahead for their own long-term care needs and think critically about their anticipated use of resources. They should ask themselves a range of questions: To what extent do my expectations or actual needs have implications for others in need of care, including long-term care? Other families? Other communities? Could I plan in such a way that I might avoid participation in the perpetuation of injustice?

Recognition has come to be understood in at least two senses: recognition of an individual's unique identity as an autonomous individual and recognition of persons as belonging to particular communities or groups. This is taken to be an essentially cognitive process wherein "there is a conscious and explicit acknowledgment of another's identity" (Gould 2007a, 250; Gould 2008). Recognition, however, should include a third dimension; namely, the recognition of others' needs for relationships, both interpersonal and associative. As Carol Gould explains it, with this third aspect "what people need is *to be in relationship*, not only to be recognized by others as being who they are" (Gould 2007, 250). Of course, our connectedness and relationships, to a great extent, constitute who we are; but the point to underscore here is our interdependence with others, not our mere membership in a community or group.

Here, then, the elderly, family caregivers, and paid caregivers are due recognition from one another. Caregivers should recognize the elderly, the elderly should recognize their caregivers, and caregivers should recognize each other. Given inequities, however, the recognition by the elderly and their family caregivers of care workers who have emigrated is most crucial for justice. The dependent elderly and their family members should recognize the identities of care workers and their need for relationship; and further, recognize that, in the case of emigrants, relationships are fragmented and carried out across great distance, threatened, and perhaps even severed.

We might add still a fourth dimension, given the conception of subjects in ecological terms: recognition of the conditions—the places—in which the elderly and others with needs for care reside and care workers provide care. When family caregivers work with long-term care institutions, for example, they should ensure that workers are not exploited and they should advocate for fair working conditions. Would-be home care workers and family members should discuss employment under conditions of respectful interaction on working conditions, pay, and benefits, and family members involved in hiring should commit to providing safe and just working conditions. In addition, given the mutually constitutive nature of identities and places, we should take care to attend to the conditions that characterize those places abroad that have shaped, and will in the future shape, who we are and will become, and that we shape with our expectations, policies, and practices.

Empathy, according to Gould, "signifies a feeling or imaginative identification with another and that other's perspective and situation" (Gould 2007a, 251). While the notions of "identification" or having "fellow feeling" (253) are ethically problematic given the profound asymmetries between the parties involved here (Young 1997), the practice of seeking knowledge of another's situation, listening carefully, and having—or at least trying to develop—feeling for the other's particular plight has value for promoting justice. At minimum, family caregivers, paid caregivers, and the elderly should cultivate what Gould calls a "disposition to empathy" (2007a, 252), which appreciates and reckons with asymmetries. Employers, health care lobbyists, and international lenders should also work to cultivate it.

As for *appreciation*, I am thinking mostly about the appreciation of family caregivers for paid care workers and appreciation on the part of the elderly for their caregivers. But we might apply it to relations between employers and employees, the loved ones of family caregivers, or the individuals in organizations that work to affix a fair "price" to care labor. Appreciation involves acknowledging the value—social and economic—of the labor provided generally and for the particular caregiver; and appreciating the consequences of the provision of the labor, both generally and for the particular caregiver, her family, and her community. Moreover, beneficiaries should explicitly and regularly express gratitude.

To speak of *solidarity* between family caregivers and paid workers, especially emigrants, is, given existing inequalities, to risk romanticizing. Still, as with recognition and empathy, there may be potential, even under conditions of asymmetry. Although differently situated, both family members and paid care workers face disrespect, financial vulnerability, job precariousness, poor health, and stress related to work and family responsibilities. Both groups, especially when we include emigrants, are embedded in the rhetoric of economic self-determination and the push toward privatized caring. These overlapping embodied, social, economic, and political conditions can serve as the basis for solidarity aimed at advancing the cause of justice, for them as well as those for whom they care.

Global solidarity, according to Kurasawa, is not only "a normative ideal or legal-institutional project from above, [it] is, just as importantly, a transnational mode of practice whereby actors construct bonds of mutual commitment and reciprocity across borders through public discourse and socio-political struggle" (160).[3] "The labour of solidarity," he suggests, "should consist of devising ways of living together that reconcile the ideals of equality and difference" (158). Gould further fleshes out the concept and practice of transnational solidarity (2007b). On her view, there is a sort of threshold element, involving "a readiness to establish broader relations with a range of others" (159), expanding beyond one's own group or community. Beyond this, solidarity includes a shared commitment to justice in addition to an affective element, a willingness "to imaginatively construct for oneself [others'] feelings and needs" (156), and a "readiness to take action" (157). Iris Young considers solidarity also to involve "a sense of commitment," but she sees it as concerning "justice owed" to others to whom we are connected in relations of injustice. While others point to the possibilities of "fellow feeling or mutual identification" in motivating solidarity, Young emphasizes the need to assume and reflect upon our asymmetries (2000, 222).

We come away, then, with a notion of solidarity as a set of practices involving reaching beyond the scope of one's regular circle to cultivate ties with others across distance and amid asymmetries— efforts to imagine what it is like for them and a willingness to stand together in advancing justice and resisting injustice. Given an ecological account of subjects, I prefer to ground solidarity in our intersubjectivity. I also want to suggest that justice need not be owed to others for us to share in practices of solidarity with them. Practices of solidarity could be organized around working conditions, reenvisioning the relationship between work and family life, cultivating respect and developing strategies to ensure adequate savings and financial security for the aged and their caregivers, access to health care, citizenship, and the equal distribution of caring labor in families. That is just for starters.

Finally, Kurasawa proposes *reciprocity* as an element of solidarity. I want to make it its own distinctive practice. Reciprocity holds that "we should return good for good, in proportion to what we receive; that we should make reparation for the harm we do; and that we should be disposed to do those things as a matter of moral obligation" (Becker 1986, 4). Reciprocity, then, calls for affluent governments, families and individuals, and the global for-profit sector to give back, and in some instances make amends. The ideas outlined above should serve as a start.

As we strive to meet our obligations to the elderly, we must resist the sort of thinking that both *under*values and at the same time *re*values care and care work to suit the needs of the well-off, that conceives of long-term care as mostly a matter of domestic (that is, state and/or personal) concern, and that suggests we can continue to lurch forward by "promulgating solutions to discrete aspects of the problem[s]" (Miller, Booth, and Mor 2008, 451).

Thinking ecologically about long-term care, responsible agents see a new social, economic, political, and ethical landscape. Here we bring into view the connectedness of policy spheres, places, and people. Indeed, we see the interdependence of: aging people in households or institutions in a particular community; family members in their own households, in workplaces, and in care settings, and paid care workers, including the growing number who are emigrants in institutional and home-based care settings, in their own homes, and perhaps, too, in border-control zones and the technologically mediated spaces that link them to distant loved ones; girls coming of age in late capitalism in care export zones; and people, including the aged and dependent, in particular low-income countries, in particular communities, struggling under particular failing health care systems and newly configured filial and communal bonds, all "interwoven in a complex, life-sustaining" or, as the case may be, life-eroding "web" (Fisher and Tronto 1990). To think ecologically is to have a method and a goal for moving forward on improving—indeed, making more equal—the conditions under and in which the elderly, their caregivers, and people needing care in source countries, become and endure. This, an ecological ethic, is the vision people should embrace collectively for just and sustainable long-term care.

Notes

Introduction

1. Like Code, I recognize liabilities that might stem from my embrace of the discourse of ecology, but opt for it anyway, finding its resources irresistible.

2. Code refers to the work of Cornelius Castoriadis on "the instituted social imaginary," which "carries within it the normative social meanings, customs, expectations, assumptions, values, prohibitions, and permissions—the habitus and ethos—into which human beings are nurtured . . . and which they internalize, affirm, challenge, or contest as they make sense of their place, options, responsibilities within a world, both social and physical, whose 'nature' and meaning are also instituted in these imaginary significations. A social imaginary is social in the broadest sense: it is not merely about principles of conduct, although it is about these too; but it is about how such principles claim and maintain salience; about the scope and limits of human knowledge and the place of knowledge in the world; about the structural ordering of institutions of knowledge production; about intellectual and moral character ideals, subjectivity, and agency; about the kinds of habitat and living conditions that are within reach and/or worth striving for; about social-political-economic organization and just distribution of goods, privileges, power, and authority. In this complex sense, the social imaginary of mastery extends across the ethos and expectations of the affluent white western world that sees no limits to human possibilities of mastering and controlling the world's resources . . . and human Others as well" (Code 2006, 30–32).

3. I make use of the terms *caregiving* and *care work* after reflection on other possibilities. I use these terms synonymously for the most part, though most often *caregiving* is used to describe the activities of family members, not paid care workers.

4. While there are important distinctions to be made between nurses and direct care workers, and among direct care workers (for instance, hospital-based nurse aides tend to earn more than those working in home care), I will discuss them largely as a group, in part because their concerns overlap to such a great extent and because "down-skilling" of nurses educated abroad is not uncommon.

Chapter One: The Plight of the Dependent Elderly and Their Families

1. For further discussion and analysis of the debate, see Institute of Medicine 2008.

2. For a history of long-term care in the United States, see Holstein and Cole 1996.

3. Important advances are being made by some companies, including geriatric care managers, to support employees, referral services, and education on how to better care for oneself as a caregiver (Dobkin 2007; Galinski, Bond, Sakai, et al., 2008). Larger nonprofits that are unionized and have more women and minorities in leadership positions tend to be the most supportive. An estimated one-fifth of companies in the United States now offer telephone resources and referral services on elder care, an increase from 15 percent in 1998. Nevertheless, some employees maintain that "they're not seeing the true picture" (Gross 2006b). Companies tend to favor strategies that cost them little or nothing; hence referral services and unpaid leaves are preferred. Meeting child care needs tends to be the prototype for many employers, reflecting a misunderstanding of long-term care needs. And for many small businesses and nonprofits, elder care benefits "seem a luxury."

4. Notably, tax law requires that consumer-directed care assistants be treated as employees rather than as self-employed and also subject to federal and state laws regarding work hours and wages, as well as workers' compensation (OECD 2005, 58).

5. Since then, Congress and the states have seen a steady flow of bills introduced for initiatives such as expansion of the FMLA to offer specific assistance to caregivers of injured as well as deployed servicemen, caregiver assessment, training, and education, care coordination, and respite care. Only a few measures have been enacted (Family Caregiver Alliance, n.d.a). Efforts to expand the population of employees eligible for the FMLA, to

pay caregivers during leave—save for those caring for veterans—have so far been unsuccessful.

Chapter Two: The Plight of Paid Workers in Long-term Care

1. Reasons for the difficulty include inconsistency over definitions of particular kinds of health workers and the fact that some migrant care workers leave under tourist or student visas and stay abroad. Analysts believe that their numbers are severely undercounted (Buchan, Parkin, and Sochalski 2003; Dumont and Zurn 2007).

2. The Commission on Graduates of Foreign Nursing Schools (CGFNS), established in 1977 by the American Nurses Association and the National League for Nursing, is responsible for reviewing educational and licensing credentials in source countries, English-language proficiency, and, for RNs, administering the CGFNS qualifying exam, taken to be a predictor of the ability to pass the NCLEX-RN exam, required by all state boards of nursing. In 1996, CGFNS launched VisaScreen to facilitate foreign-educated nurses' ability to meet government requirements for visas. The Illegal Immigration Reform and Immigrant Responsibility Act, (1996) demands screening prior to visas being issued to health care professionals educated abroad (Commission on Graduates of Foreign Nursing Schools 2010).

Chapter Three: Tracing Injustice in Long-term Care

1. Giorgio Agamben's work on Foucault's concept of an "apparatus" may be helpful here. An apparatus, he writes, is "literally anything that has in some way the capacity to capture, orient, determine, intercept, model, control, or secure the gestures, behaviors, opinions, or discourses of living beings." Invoked in "investigation of concrete modes in which the positivities (or the apparatuses) act within the relations, mechanisms, and 'plays' of power," an apparatus is "the network [le reseau] that can be established between these elements" (2009, 6–7).

2. Recruiters, indeed, are said to select particular areas on the basis of particular "representations of people and places" (Tyner 1996, 413).

3. See Frye 1983.

4. The literature on the concept of exploitation is extensive. Frye's analysis is one among many.

5. This is difficult to measure. Studies estimate that developing coun-

tries received more than $140 billion in 2004, a 57 percent increase over 2001 (World Bank 2004). Some estimate that unrecorded remittances may have amounted to more than $50 billion in 2004 (Page and Plaza 2006). Latin America, East Asia, and the Pacific garnered the greatest share in 2004, with significant increases in South Asia. At the country level, while India, Mexico, the Philippines, and Egypt once led in remittance receipts, in 2005 China became the leader. Latin America, the Middle East, and North Africa received the largest remittances per capita. In South Asia, the Middle East, and North Africa, this income constitutes a substantial share of GDP (Page and Plaza 2006). There are, not surprisingly, problems with these data. The IMF, for instance, publishes data on workers' remittances, but the data are not comprehensively reported and fail to account for transfers that take place in informal channels (Page and Plaza 2006). Researchers have called for efforts to disaggregate remittances into different types (e.g., family, collective, and entrepreneurial) and explore gender differences in order to garner more accurate data on their impact (Sørenson 2005b).

6. For a review of current health indicators for the Philippines, see www.who.int/countries/phl/en/.

7. For health indicators for Jamaica see www.who.int/countries/jam/en/.

8. For health indicators for India see www.who.int/countries/ind/en/.

Chapter Four: An Ecological Ethic

1. The prevailing liability conception of responsibility emphasizes a different sort of relationship wherein direct harms are perpetrated by identifiable agents on particular others. See the discussion in Young 2006.

2. Tronto refers to children in her remarks.

3. Nussbaum's theory is especially noteworthy for being the only one to explicitly address care labor (2006, 170–212). She notably cites as her eighth principle of justice that care for children, the ill, and the elderly "should be a prominent focus of the world community" given its essential role in nurturing people's capabilities (321). Nussbaum further argues that when it comes to care, the policy issue has two "faces": the cared-for (children and adults with disabilities) and the lives of those who care for them (usually adults, and most often women, both related and unrelated, paid and unpaid); and it has three "locations": the public sector, the educational system, and the workplace (212). State-centered, Nussbaum's account

makes a place for a "thin, decentralized global structure of responsibility" (314) that includes domestic structures along with international bodies.

Nussbaum is surely right to include this among her principles of justice and also to include a role for place. Yet there is more to be said about these faces and locations. Within the scope of concern here, indeed, are the cared-for and the carers, yet the latter group includes not just family and nonfamily members offering unpaid assistance but also both native and emigrant care workers engaged in paid care work. Moreover, there are people who need care but cannot get it due to the absence of health workers in their communities, a circumstance increasingly attributable to migration. We could also include families of emigrant care workers. There are ultimately seven general (intersecting) "locations" of interest: the public sector, the educational system, homes, and the workplace, as well as the settings where care is provided, public and private, the places where it is needed but not available, and finally, transnational space, linking and separating places and traversed by migrants in body and imagination. Nussbaum's account obscures the implications of the transnational structure of care, including long-term care, work. Given the magnitude of the current worldwide need for care and the cross-border flows of care workers from places with precariously propped health systems to ones replete with resources, her account also undertheorizes the relationship between locations. In the next chapter I argue that more robust global structures of responsibility are necessary. There is also a vital role for individuals, not just states and institutions.

4. I grant that there may be pejorative connotations with the concept *enduring*. Here I hope to avoid the association of surviving unrelenting hardship.

5. Nussbaum's solution is to embrace a more Aristotelian, less Kantian image of the person, "bringing the rational and the animal into a more intimate relation with one another, [thus] acknowledging that there are many types of dignity in the world" (54). An ecological account, however, highlights embodiment, temporality, and the relationality and locatedness (structurally and spatially) of subjects as central to understanding and addressing injustice.

6. The argument here bears a family resemblance to the conception of the person put forward by ecological feminism. See Cuomo 1998.

7. I am grateful to Ryoa Chung and Christine Straehle for their help in formulating this line of argument.

Chapter Five: Realizing Justice Globally in Long-term Care

1. Here I combine the insights of O'Neill (2000) and Young (2006) regarding parameters of responsibility. I agree with O'Neill that capacity is important, but with Young want to maintain that all agents have some capacity, and, moreover, to home in more precisely on the relationship between agents and victims of injustice.

2. For fuller discussion of the array of options and analysis, see Packer, Labonté, and Spitzer 2007.

3. Solidarity has traditionally been theorized as concerning relations between members of a particular group, region, or society. See, for example, Dean 1996 and Bayertz 1999.

References

AARP. 2008. Valuing the Invaluable: The Economic Value of Family Caregiving, 2008 update. Washington, DC: AARP.

AARP International. 2008. International Day of Older Persons 2008: Global Perspectives on Family Caregiving. Executive Summary. Washington, DC: AARP.

Abelson, R. 2002. Bringing discipline (and scorecards) to nursing homes. *New York Times*, July 7.

Abraham, B. 2004. Women Nurses and the Notion of Their "Empowerment." Discussion paper no. 88, Kerala Research Programme on Local Level Development Centre for Development Studies, Thiruvananthapuram.

Academy Health. 2008. Voluntary Code of Ethical Conduct for the Recruitment of Foreign-Educated Nurses to the United States. Washington, DC: Academy Health.

Acosta, P., Calderon, C., Fajnzylber, P., and Lopez, H. 2008. What is the impact of international remittances on poverty and inequality in Latin America? *World Development* 36 (1): 89–114.

Adams, A. 2004. Remittances and Poverty in Guatamala. World Bank Policy Research Working Paper no. 3418. Washington, DC: World Bank.

Adlung, R. 2002. Health services in a globalising world. *Eurohealth* 8 (3): 18–21.

AFL-CIO. N.d. Family and medical leave. Available at www.aflcio.org/issues/workfamily/fmla.cfm (accessed March 5, 2010).

Agamben, G. 2009. What Is an Apparatus? And Other Essays. Stanford: Stanford University Press.

Agency for Healthcare Research and Quality. 2000. Long-term Care Users Range in Age and Most Do Not Live in Nursing Homes: Research Alert. Rockville, MD: AHRQ.

Ahmad, O. B. 2005. Managing medical migration from poor countries. *British Medical Journal* 331: 43–45.

Aiken, L. H. 2007. US nurse labor market dynamics are key to global nurse sufficiency. *Health Services Research* 42 (3 pt. 2): 1299–320.

Aiken, L. H., Clarke, S. P., Stone, D. M., Sochalski, J. A., Busse, R., Clark, H., Giovannetti, P. . . . and Shamian, J. 2001. Nurses' reports on hospital care in five countries. *Health Affairs* 20 (3): 43–53.

Akintola, O. 2004. A Gendered Analysis of the Burden of Care on Family and Volunteer Caregivers in Uganda and South Africa. Durban: HEARD.

Alcaron-Gonzalez, D. and McKinley, T. 1999. The adverse effects of structural adjustment on working women in Mexico. *Latin American Perspectives* 26: 103–17.

Allan, H., and Larsen, J. A. 2003. "We Need Respect": Experiences of Internationally Recruited Nurses in the UK. London: Royal College of Nursing.

Alliance for Aging Research (AAR). 2003. Ageism: How Health Care Fails the Elderly. Washington, DC: AAR.

Alonso-Garbayo, A., and Maben, J. 2009. Internationally recruited nurses from India and the Philippines in the United Kingdom: The decision to emigrate. *Human Resources for Health* 7: 37.

Alzheimer's Association. 2007. Alzheimer's Disease Facts and Figures. Chicago, IL: Alzheimer's Association.

American Geriatrics Society. 2009. ADGAP surveys of geriatric medicine fellowship programs—2009 update. New York: AGS.

American Hospital Association. 2007. The 2007 State of America's Hospitals. Washington, DC: AHA.

Anand S., and Bärnighausen, T. 2004. Human resources and health outcomes: Cross-country econometric study. *Lancet* 364: 1603–9.

Anderson, B., and Isaacs, A. A. 2007. Simply not there: The impact of international migration of nurses and midwives—Perspectives from Guyana. *Journal of Midwifery and Women's Health* 52 (4): 392–97.

Anderson, G., and Horvath, J. 2004. The growing burden of chronic disease in America. *Public Health Reports* 119 (3): 263–70.

———. 2002. Chronic Conditions: Making the Case for Ongoing Care. Baltimore: Johns Hopkins University Press.

Arends-Kuenning, M. 2006. The balance of care: Trends in the wages and employment of immigrant nurses in the US between 1990 and 2000. *Globalizations* 3 (September): 333–48.

Arno, P. S. 2006. Economic value of family caregiving: 2004. Paper presented at Care Coordination and Caregiver Forum. Bethesda, MD, January 25–27.

Asch, A., Blustein, J., and Wasserman, D. T. 2008. Criticizing and reforming segregated facilities for persons with disabilities. *Journal of Bioethical Inquiry* 5: 157–67.

Asch, S. M., Kerr, E. A., Joan, K., Adams, J., Setodji, C. M., Malik, S., and McGlynn, E. A. 2006. Who is at greatest risk for receiving poor quality health care? *New England Journal of Medicine* 354 (11): 1147–56.

Association of Directors of Geriatric Academic Programs (ADGAP). 2004. Financial compensation for geriatricians in academic and private practice. *Training and Practice Update* 2 (2): 1–7.

Awumbila, M., and Ardayfio-Schandorf, E. 2008. Gendered poverty, migration, and livelihood strategies of female porters in Accra, Ghana. *Norwegian Journal of Geography* 62: 171–79.

Bach, S. 2010. Managed migration? Nurse recruitment and the consequences of state policy. *Industrial Relations Journal* 41 (3): 249–66.

———. 2003. International Migration of Health Workers: Labour and Social Issues. Geneva: International Labour Organisation.

Bachu, A., and O'Connell, M. 2001. Fertility of American Women, Current Population Report P20-543RV. Washington, DC: U.S. Census Bureau.

Badgett, L., and Folbre, N. 1999. Assigning care: Gender norms and economic outcomes. *International Labour Review* 138 (3): 311–26.

Baldock, C. V. 2000. Migrants and their parents: Caregiving from a distance. *Journal of Family Issues* 21: 205–24.

Ball, M. M., Perkins, M. M., Whittington, F. J., Connell, B. R., Hollingsworth, C., King, S. V., Elrod, C. L., and Combs, B. L. 2004. Managing decline in assisted living: The key to aging in place. *Journal of Gerontology Series B: Psychological Services and Social Sciences* 59 (4): S202–S12.

Ball, R. E. 2008. Globalised labour markets and the trade of Filipino nurses. In J. Connell, ed., The International Migration of Health Workers. New York: Routledge.

———. 2004. Divergent development, racialised rights: Globalised labour markets and the trade of nurses—the case of the Philippines. *Women's Studies International Forum* 27: 119–33.

—————. 2000. The individual and global processes: Labor migration decision making and Filipino nurses. *Pilipinas* 34: 63–92.

Ball, R. E., and Piper, N. 2002. Globalisation and regulation of citizenship: Filipino migrant workers in Japan. *Political Geography* 21: 1013–34.

Barber, P. G. 2009. Border contradictions and the reproduction of gender and class inequalities in Philippine global migration. Paper presented at International Studies Association, New York, New York, February 17.

—————. 2000. Agency in Philippine women's labour migration and provisional diaspora. *Women's Studies International Forum* 23 (4): 399–411.

Bayertz, K. 1999. Four uses of solidarity. In K. Bayertz, ed., Solidarity. Dordrecht: Kluwer.

Beine, M., Docquier, F., and Rapaport, H. 2001. Brain drain and economic growth: Theory and evidence. *Journal of Development Economics* 64 (1): 275–89.

Beneria, H. 1999. Globalization, gender, and the Davos Man. *Feminist Economics* 5 (3): 61–83.

Bergson, H. 1911. Creative Evolution. New York: Henry Holt. Translated by Arthur Mitchell.

Berliner, H. S., and Ginzberg, E. 2002. Why this hospital nursing shortage is different. *JAMA* 288 (21): 2742–44.

Better Jobs Better Care. 2007. Respectful relationships: The heart of better jobs better care. BJBC Issue Brief no. 7.

—————. 2005. Family care and paid care: Separate worlds or common ground? BJBC Issue Brief no. 5.

—————. 2004. Health insurance coverage for direct care workers: Riding out the storm. BJBC Issue Brief no. 3.

Bettio, F., Simonazzi, A., and Villa, P. 2006. Changes in care regimes and female migration: The "care drain" in the Mediterranean. *Journal of European Social Policy* 16 (3): 271–85.

Biggs, S., and Powell, J. L. 2001. A Foucauldian analysis of old age and the power of social welfare. *Journal of Aging and Social Policy* 12 (2): 93–112.

Boockvar, K., Fishman, E., Kyriacou, C. K., Monias, A., Gavi, S., and Cortes, T. 2004. Adverse events due to discontinuations in drug use and dose changes in patients transferred between acute and long-term care facilities. *Archives of Internal Medicine* 164 (5): 545–50.

Bosniak, L. 2009. Citizenship, non-citizenship, and the transnationalization of domestic work. In S. Benhabib and J. Resnik, eds., Migrations and Mobilities: Citizenship, Borders, and Gender. New York: New York University Press.

Bowers, B. J., Esmond, S., and Jacobson, N. 2003. Turnover reinterpreted: CNAs talk about why they leave. *Journal of Gerontological Nursing* 29 (3): 36–43.

Brannon, D., Barry, T., Kemper, P., Schreiner, A., and Vasey, J. 2007. Job perceptions and intent to leave among direct care workers: Evidence from the Better Jobs Better Care demonstrations. *Gerontologist* 47 (6): 820–29.

Brown, E. A. 2008. The Jamaican experience with the movement of natural persons. Paper presented at WTO Symposium on GATS Mode 4. Geneva, 22–23 September.

Brown, R., Peikes, D., Chen, A., Ng, J., Schore, J., and Soh, C. 2007. The Evaluation of the Medicare Coordinated Policy Demonstration: Findings for the First Two Years. Washington, DC: Mathematica Policy Research.

Browne, C., and Braun, K. L. 2008. Globalization, women's migration, and the long-term care workforce. *Gerontologist* 48 (1): 16–24.

Brush, B. L. 1995. The Rockefeller agenda for American/Philippines nursing relations. *Western Journal of Nursing Research* 17 (5): 540–55.

———. 1993. "Exchanges" or employees? The exchange visitors program and foreign nurse immigration to the United States, 1945–1990. *Nursing History Review* 1: 171–80.

Brush, B. L., and Sochalski, J. 2007. International nurse migration: Lessons from the Philippines. *Policy, Politics, and Nursing Practice* 8: 37–46.

Brush, B., and Vaspurum, V. 2006. Nurses, nannies, and caring work: Importation, visibility, and marketability. *Nursing Inquiry* 13: 181–85.

Buchan, J., Parkin, T., Sochalski, J. 2003. *International Nurse Mobility: Trends and Policy Implications*. Geneva: WHO.

Bundred, P. E., and Levitt C. 2000. Medical migration: Who are the real losers? *Lancet* 356: 245–46.

Bussolo, M., and Medvedev, D. 2007. Do Remittances Have a Flip Side? A General Equilibrium Analysis of Remittances, Labor Supply Responses, and Policy Options for Jamaica. World Bank Policy Research Working Paper no. 4143 (March).

Cannuscio, C. C., Jones, C., Kawachi, I., Colditz, G. A., Berkman, L., and Rimm, E. 2002. Reverberations of family illness: A longitudinal assessment of informal caregiving and mental health status in the nurses' health study. *American Journal of Public Health* 92 (8): 1305–11.

Carers UK. 2009. Business leaders offer help to employers to mitigate recession. Available at www.carersuk.org/Newsandcampaigns/News/1233068607 (accessed October 28, 2010).

Carers UK and Centre for Social Inclusion, Sheffield Hallam University. 2006. Who Cares Wins: The Social and Business Benefits of Supporting Working Carers. Available at www.carersuk.org/Policyandpractice/Research/Employmentandcaring (accessed October 28, 2010).

CARICOM/PAHO. 2005. Report of the Caribbean Commission on Health and Development. St. Lucia: CARICOM/PAHO.

Cartier, C. 2003. From home to hospital and back again: Economic restructuring, end of life, and the gendered problems of place-switching health services. *Social Science and Medicine* 56 (11): 2289–301.

Carr, M., Chen, M. A., and Tate, J. 2000. Globalization and home-based workers. *Feminist Economics* 6 (3): 123–42.

Casey, E. S. 1999. The tie of the glance: Toward becoming otherwise. In E. Grosz, ed., Becomings: Explorations in Time, Memory, and Futures. Ithaca, NY: Cornell University Press.

———. 1997. The Fate of Place: A Philosophical History. Berkeley: University of California Press.

Castle, N. G., Engberg, J., Anderson, R., and Men, A. 2007. Job satisfaction of nurse aides in nursing homes: Intent to leave and turnover. *Gerontologist* 47 (2): 193–204.

Center for Worklife Law. 2008. Addressing Family Responsibility Discrimination. Policy Briefing Series, Issue 16. Hastings: University of California-Hastings Center for Worklife Law.

Centers for Medicare and Medicaid Services. 2002. Appropriateness of Minimum Nurse Staffing Ratios in Nursing Homes: Phase II Final Report. Baltimore: Centers for Medicare and Medicaid Services.

Chaguturu S., and Vallabhaneni, S. 2005. Aiding and abetting: Nursing crises at home and abroad. *New England Journal of Medicine* 353 (17): 1761–63.

Chami, R., Fullenkamp, C., and Jahjah, S. 2005. Are Immigrant Remittance Flows a Source of Capital for Development? IMF Staff Papers 52, 1.

Chant, S., and McIlwaine, C. 1995. Women of a Lesser Cost: Female Labour, Foreign Exchange, and Philippine Development. London: Pluto.

Chatterjee, P. 2010. Progress patchy on health worker crisis. *Lancet* 377: 456.

Chen, L., Evans, T., Anand, S., Boufford, J. I., Brown, H., Chowdhury, M. . . . and Wibulpolprasert, S. 2004. Human resources for health: Overcoming the crisis. *Lancet* 364: 1984–90.

Cheung, R., and Aiken, L. H. 2006. Hospital initiatives to support a better-educated workforce. *Journal of Nursing Administration* 36 (7–8): 357–62.

Choy, C. C. 2003. Empire of Care: Nursing and Migration in Filipino American History. Durham, NC: Duke University Press.

Christakis, N. A., and Allison, P. D. 2006. Mortality after the hospitalization of a spouse. *New England Journal of Medicine* 354 (7): 719–30.

Christopherson, S. 2006. Women and the restructuring of care work: Cross national variations and trends in ten OECD countries. In M. K. Zimmerman, J. S. Litt, and C. E. Bose, eds., Global Dimensions of Gender and Carework. Stanford, CA: Stanford Social Sciences.

Cigolle, C. T., Langa, K. M., Kabeto, M. U., and Blaum, C. S. 2007. Geriatric conditions and disability: The health and retirement study. *Annals of Internal Medicine* 147 (3): 156.

Cock, K. M., and Weiss, H. A. 2000. The global epidemiology of HIV/AIDS. *Tropical Medicine and International Health* 5 (7): A3–9.

Code, L. 2006. Ecological Knowing: The Politics of Epistemic Location. Oxford: Oxford University Press.

Commodore, V. R., Devereaux, P. J., Zhou, Q., Stone, S. B., Busse, J. W., Ravindran, N. C., Burns K. . . . and Guyatt, G. 2009. Quality of care in for-profit and not-for-profit nursing homes: Systematic review and meta-analysis. *British Medical Journal* 339: 2732.

Congressional Research Service. 2009. Leave Benefits in the United States.

Conley, V. A. 1997. Ecopolitics: The Environment in Poststructuralist Thought. London: Routledge.

Connell, J., and Brown, R. P. C. 2004. The remittances of migrant Tongan and Samoan nurses from Australia. *Human Resources for Health* 2 (2): 1–21.

Connell, J., and Stilwell, B. 2006. Recruiting agencies in the global health care chain. In C. Kuptsch, ed., Merchants of Labour. Geneva: ILO.

Council on Graduates of Foreign Nursing Schools. 2010. Immigration and visas: Frequently asked questions. Available at www.cgfns.org/sections/tools/faq/imm.shtml (accessed November 10, 2010).

Covinsky, K. E., Eng, C., Lui, L.-Y., Sands, L. P., Sehgal, A. R., Walter, L. C. . . . and Yaffe, K. 2001. Reduced employment in caregivers of frail elders: Impact of ethnicity, patient clinical characteristics, and caregiver characteristics. *Journals of Gerontology: Medical Sciences* 56 (11): M707–M713.

Coward, S. 2007. CARICOM: Mass migration of Caribbean professionals cause for concern (17 May). Available at www.caribbeanpressreleases .com/articles/1796/1/CARICOM-Mass-Migration-of-Caribbean-Profes sionals-Cause-for-Concern/Page1/html (accessed June 10, 2009).

Cuomo, C. 1998. Feminism and Ecological Communities: An Ethic of Flourishing. New York: Routledge.

Dalla Costa, M., and Dalla Costa, G. 1995. Paying the Price: Women and The Politics of International Economic Strategy. London: Zed Books.

Daly, M., ed. 2001. Care Work: The Quest for Security. Geneva: ILO.

Dauvergne, C. 2009. Globalizing fragmentation: New pressures on women caught in the immigration law-citizenship law dichotomy. In S. Benhabib and J. Resnik, eds., Migrations and Mobilities: Citizenship, Borders, and Gender. New York: New York University Press.

Dawson, S. 2003. Long-term Care Financing and the Long-term Care Workforce Crisis: Causes and Solutions. Washington, DC: Citizens for Long Term Care.

Dean, J. 1996. Solidarity of Strangers. Berkeley: University of California Press.

Decker, F. H., Gruhn, P., Matthews-Martin, L., Dollard, K. J., Tucker, A. M., and Bizette, L. 2003. 2002 AHCA Survey of Nursing Staff Vacancy and Turnover in Nursing Homes. Washington, DC: American Health Care Association.

Deeb-Sossa, N., and Mendez, J. B. 2008. Enforcing borders in the Nuevo South: Gender and migration in Williamsburg, Virginia and the Research Triangle, North Carolina. *Gender and Society* 22 (October): 613–38.

de Voelker, R. 2010. Ethnic shifts raise issues in elder care. *JAMA* 303 (4): 321.

DiCicco-Bloom, B. 2004. The racial and gendered experiences of immigrant nurses from Kerala, India. *Journal of Transcultural Nursing* 15: 26–33.

Direct Care Alliance. 2005. Issue brief 3: A poorly trained paraprofessional workforce. Available at www.directcarealliance.org/sections/pubs/Issue Brief3.htm (accessed July 14, 2008).

Dobkin, L. 2007. How to confront the elder care challenge. Workforce Management Online (April). Available at www.workforce.com/section/09/feature/24/85/10/index.html (accessed March 5, 2010).

Docquier, F., Lowell, B. L., and Marfouk, A. 2007. A Gendered Assessment of the Brain Drain. Discussion Paper no. 3235. Bonn: IZA.

Domingues, D. S. M., and Postel-Vinay, F. 2003. Migration as a source of growth: The perspective of a developing country. *Journal of Population Economics* 16 (1): 161–75.

Donelan, K., Hill, C. A., Hoffman, C., Scoles, K., Feldman, P. H., Levine, C., and Gould, D. 2002. Challenged to care: Informal caregivers in a changing health system. *Health Affairs* 21 (4): 222–31.

Doty, P. 2004. Consumer-directed home care: Effects on family caregivers. Policy Brief. Family Caregiver Alliance. Washington, DC: Family Caregiver Alliance.

Dumont, J.-C., and Zurn, P. 2007. Immigrant health workers in OECD countries in the broader context of highly skilled migration. In International Migration Outlook. Paris: OECD.

Dumont, J.-C., Martin J. P., and Spielvogel, G. 2007. Women on the Move: The Neglected Gender Dimension of the Brain Drain. IZA Discussion Paper no. 2920. Bonn.

Eaton, L. 2002. Elderly need better-coordinated services to keep them independent. *British Medical Journal* 325: 988.

Eckenwiler, L. 2009. The WHO Code on the Recruitment of International Health Personnel: We've only just begun. *Developing World Bioethics* 9 (1): ii–v.

Economic Commission for Latin America and the Caribbean (ECLAC). 2006a. Emigration of Nurses from the Caribbean: Causes and Consequences for the Socio-economic Welfare of the Country: Trinidad and Tobago—A Case Study. Port of Spain, Trinidad and Tobago: ECLAC.

———. 2006b. Migration in the Caribbean—What Do We Know? An Overview of Data, Policies, and Programmes at the International and Regional Levels to Address Critical Issues. Port of Spain: Trinidad and Tobago: ECLAC.

———. 2004. Population Ageing in the Caribbean: Longevity and Quality of Life. Port of Spain: Trinidad and Tobago: ECLAC.

————. 2003. The Brain Drain in the Health Sector: Emigration of Nurses from Trinidad and Tobago—A Case Study. Port of Spain: Trinidad and Tobago: ECLAC.

Ehrenreich, B., and Hochschild, A. R., eds. 2002. Global Woman: Nannies, Maids, and Sex Workers in the New Economy. New York: Henry Holt.

Emanuel, E. J., Fairclough, D. L., Slutsman, J., and Emanuel, L. 2000. Understanding economic and other burdens of terminal illness: The experience of patients and their caregivers. *Annals of Internal Medicine* 132 (6): 451–59.

Escrivá, A. 2004. Securing Care and Welfare of Dependents Transnationally: Peruvians and Spaniards in Spain. Oxford: Oxford Institute of Ageing Working Papers. Oxford: Oxford Institute of Population Aging.

Ettner, S. L. 1995. The impact of "parent care" on female labor supply decisions. *Demography* 32 (1): 63–80.

Eyal, N., and Hurst, S. 2008. Brain drain: Is nothing to be done? *Journal of Public Health Ethics* 1 (2): 180–92.

Faini, R. 2003. The Brain Drain: An Unmitigated Blessing? Centro Studi Luca d'Agliano Development Studies Working Paper no. 173.

————. 2001. Development, Trade, and Migration. International Monetary Fund.

Family Caregiver Alliance (FCA). N.d.a. Federal and state family caregiving legislation: A summary of bills from 2004–2006. Available at www .fca.org (accessed July 13, 2008).

————. N.d.b. Policy and advocacy. Available at www.caregiver.org/caregiver/jsp (accessed July 13, 2008).

Fang, Z. Z. 2007. Potential of China in global nurse migration. *Health Services Research* 42 (3):1419–28.

Federal Interagency Forum on Aging-Related Statistics. 2006. Older Americans Update 2006: Key Indicators of Well-Being. Washington, DC: U.S. Government Printing Office.

Feinberg, L. F., and Newman, S. L. 2006. Preliminary experiences of the states in implementing the National Family Caregiver Support Program: A 50 state study. *Journal of Aging and Social Policy* 3 (4): 95–113.

Fisher, B., and Tronto, J. 1990. Toward a feminist theory of caring. In E. K. Abel and M. K. Nelson, eds., Circles of Care: Work and Identity in Women's Lives. Albany: SUNY Press.

Fleming, K. C., Evans, J. M., and Chutka, D. S. 2003. Caregiver and clinician shortages in an aging nation. *Mayo Clinic Proceedings* 78 (8): 1026–40.

Folbre, N. 2006. Demanding quality: Worker/consumer coalitions and "high road" strategies in the care sector. *Politics and Society* 34 (1): 11–31.

———. 2001. The Invisible Heart: Economics and Family Values. New York: New Press.

———. 1999. The Invisible Heart: Care and the Global Economy. In Human Development Report. New York: United Nations Development Program.

Folbre, N., and Nelson, J. A. 2000. For love or money—or both? *Journal of Economic Perspectives* 14 (94): 123–40.

Fouron, G., and Glick-Schiller, N. 2001. All in the family: Gender, transnational migration, and the nation-state. *Identities: Global Studies in Culture and Power* 7 (4): 539–82.

Foust, J. B., Naylor, M. D., Boling, P. A., and Cappuzzo, K. A. 2005. Opportunities for improving post-hospital home medication management among older adults. *Home Health Services Quarterly* 24 (102): 101–22.

Fraser, N. 2009. Scales of Justice: Reimagining Political Space in a Globalizing World. New York: Columbia University Press.

Frye, M. 1983. The Politics of Reality: Essays in Feminist Theory. Freedom, CA: Crossing Press.

Fussel, E. 2000. Making labor flexible: The recomposition of Tijuana's maquiladora female labor force. *Feminist Economics* 6 (3): 59–79.

Galinski, E., Bond, J. T., Sakai, K., Kim, S. S., and Giuntoli, N. 2008. 2008 National Study of Employers. New York: Families and Work Institute.

Garland-Thomson, R. 2010. What can disability studies do for bioethics? Paper presented at International Network for Feminist Approaches to Bioethics, Singapore, July 26–28.

Genosko, G. 2009. Subjectivity and art in Guatarri's The Three Ecologies. In B. Herzogenrath, ed., Deleuze, Guattari and Ecology. New York: Palgrave Macmillan.

George, A. 2007. Human Resources for Health: A Gender Analysis. Paper prepared for the Women and Gender Equity, and Health Systems Knowledge Networks of the WHO Commission on the Social Determinants of Health. Available at www.sarpn.org.za/documents/d0002790/HR_health_George_Jul2007.pdf (accessed October 29, 2008).

Gerein, N., Green, A., and Pearson, S. 2006. The implications of shortages of health personnel for maternal health in sub-Saharan Africa. *Repro-ductive Health Matters* 14: 40–50.

Gerson, J., Oliver, T., Gutierrez, C., and Ranji, U. 2005. Addressing the Nursing Shortage. Washington, DC: Kaiser Family Foundation.

Gibson, M. J., and Houser, A. 2007. Valuing the Invaluable: A New Look at the Economic Value of Family Caregiving. Washington, DC: AARP.

Glenn, E. N. 2006. From unequal freedom: How gender and race shaped American citizenship and labor. In M. K. Zimmerman, J. S. Litt, and C. E. Bose, eds., Global Dimensions of Gender and Carework. Stanford, CA: Stanford University Press.

———. 1992. From servitude to service work: Historical continuities in the racial division of paid reproductive labor. *Signs* 18 (Autumn): 1–43.

Go, S. 2003. Recent trends in migration movements and policies: The movement of Filippino professionals and managers. In S. Go, Migration and the Labour Market in Asia. Paris: OECD.

Godfrey, J. R., and Warshaw, G. A. 2009. Toward optimal health: Considering the enhanced healthcare needs of women caregivers. *Journal of Women's Health* 18 (11): 1739–42.

Gokhale, S. D. 2007. Health and aging in India. In M. Robinson, W. Novelli, C. Pearson, L. Norris, eds., Health and Global Aging. San Francisco: Jossey-Bass.

Goldring, L. 2001. The gender and cartography of citizenship in Mexico-US transnational spaces. *Identities: Global Studies in Culture and Power* 7 (4): 501–37.

———. 2003. Gender, status and the state in transnational spaces: The gendering of political participation and Mexican hometown associations. In P. Hondagneu-Sotelo, ed., Gendered Transitions: Mexican Experiences of Immigration. Berkeley, CA: University of California.

Goldsteen, M., Abma, T., Oesburg, B., Verkerk, M., Verhey, F., and Widdershoven, G. 2007. What is it to be a daughter? Identities under pressure in dementia care. *Bioethics* 21 (1): 1–12.

Gordon, S. 2005. Nursing against the Odds: How Health Care Cost-Cutting, Media Stereotypes, and Medical Hubris Undermine Nurses and Patient Care. Ithaca: Cornell University Press.

Gould, C. C. 2009. Reconceiving autonomy and universality as norms for transnational democracy. In A. Langlois and K. Soltan, eds., Global Democracy and Its Difficulties. London: Routledge.

———. 2008. Recognition in redistribution: Care and diversity in global justice. *Southern Journal of Philosophy* 46: 91–103.

———. 2007a. Recognition, empathy, and solidarity. In G. W. Bertram, R. Celikates, C. Laudou, and D. Lauer, eds., Socialité et Reconnaissance. Grammaires de l'Humain. Paris: Editions L'Harmattan.

———. 2007b. Transnational solidarities. *Journal of Social Philosophy* 38 (1): 148–64.

Graham, H. 2010. Where is the future in public health? *Milbank Quarterly* 88 (2): 149–68.

Gross, J. 2007. New options (and risks) in home care for elderly. *New York Times,* March 1.

———. 2006a. Geriatrics lags in an age of high tech medicine. *New York Times*, October 18.

———. 2006b. As parents age, baby boomers and business struggle to cope. *New York Times*, March 25.

———. 2006c. Elder care costs deplete savings of a generation. *New York Times*, December 30.

Grosz, E. 2005. Time Travels: Feminism, Nature, Power. Durham, NC: Duke University Press.

———. 1999. Thinking the New: Of Futures Yet Unthought. In E. Grosz, ed., Becomings: Explorations in Time, Memory, and Futures. Ithaca, NY: Cornell University Press.

———. 1995. Space, Time, and Perversion: Essays on the Politics of Bodies. New York: Routledge.

Gupta, S., Pattillo, C. A., and Wagh, S. 2009. Effect of remittances on poverty and financial development in sub-Saharan Africa. *World Development* 37 (1): 104–15.

Guterman, S. 2007. Enhancing value in Medicare: Chronic care initiatives to improve the program. Testimony before the US Senate Special Committee on Aging (9 May).

Halford, S., Savage, M., and Witz, A. 1997. Genders, Careers and Organisations: Current Developments in Banking, Nursing, and Local Government. London: Macmillan.

Harmuth, S. 2002. The direct care workforce crisis in long-term care. *North Carolina Medical Journal* 63 (2): 87–94.

Harper, S., Aboderin, I., and Ruchieva, I. 2008. The impact of the out-migration of female care workers on informal family care in Nigeria and Bulgaria. In J. Connell, ed., The International Migration of Health Workers. New York: Routledge.

Harrington, C., and Pollock, A. M. 1998. Decentralisation and privatization of long-term care in the UK and USA. *Lancet* 351: 1805–8.

Harvath, T. A., Swafford, K., Smith, K., Miller, L. L., Volpin, M., Sexson, K. . . . and Young, H. A. 2008. Enhancing nursing leadership in long-term care. *Research in Gerontological Nursing* 1 (3): 187–96.

Healey, M. 2006. Outsourcing Care: Ethics and Consequences of the Global Trade in Indian Nurses. Available at www.sueztosuva.org.au/south_asia/2006?Healey.pdf (accessed July 14, 2008).

Heinrich, J. 2001. Nursing Workforce: Multiple Factors Create Nurse Recruitment and Retention Problems, Report no. GAO-01-912T. Washington, DC: US General Accounting Office (GAO).

Hernes, H. M. 2006. Woman-friendly states and a public culture of care. In M. K. Zimmerman, J. S. Litt, and C. E. Bose, eds., Global Dimensions of Gender and Carework. Stanford, CA: Stanford Social Sciences.

Heyman, J., Earle, A., and Hayes, J. 2007. The Work, Family, and Equity Index: How Does the United States Measure Up? Montreal: Institute for Health and Social Policy, McGill University.

Hildrebrandt, N., and McKenzie, D. 2006. The Effects of Migration on Child Health in Mexico. World Bank Policy Working Paper no. 3573. Washington, DC: World Bank.

Hochschild, A. R. 2002. Love and Gold. In B. Ehrenreich and A. R. Hochschild, eds., Nannies, Maids, and Sex Workers in the New Economy. New York: Henry Holt.

———. 2000. Global care chains and emotional surplus value. In W. Hutton and A. Giddens, eds., On the Edge: Living with the Global Capitalism. London: Jonathan Cape.

Holden, C. 2002. The internationalization of long-term care provision: Economics and strategy. *Global Social Policy* 2 (1): 47–67.

Holstein, M., and Cole, T. R. 1996. The evolution of long-term care in America. In R. H. Binstock, L. E. Cluff, and O. Von Mering, eds., The Future of Long-term Care: Social and Policy Issues. Baltimore: Johns Hopkins University Press.

Hondagneu-Sotelo, P., and E. Avila. 1997. "I'm here, but I'm not here": The meanings of Latina transnational motherhood. *Gender and Society* 11 (5): 548–71.

Hoppe, R. 2005. Looking Abroad to Meet the Demands for Caregivers. Washington, DC: AARP Global Aging Program.

Ilcan, S., Oliver, M., and O'Connor, D. 2007. Spaces of governance: Gender and public sector restructuring in Canada. *Gender, Place, and Culture: A Journal of Feminist Geography* 14 (10): 71–92.

Inouye, S. K., Studenski, S., Tinetti, M. E., and Kuchel., G. A. 2007. Geriatric syndromes: Clinical, research, and policy implications of a core geriatric concept. *Journal of the American Geriatrics Society* 55 (5): 780–91.

Institute of Ecosystem Studies. N.d. Definition of "ecology." Available at www.ecostudies.org/definition_ecology.html (accessed June 12, 2009).

Institute of Medicine. 2008. Retooling for an Aging America. Washington, DC: National Academies Press.

———. 2003. Keeping Patients Safe: Transforming the Work Environment of Nurses. Washington, DC: National Academies Press.

———. 2001a. Improving the Quality of Long-Term Care. Washington, DC: National Academies Press.

———. 2001b. Crossing the Quality Chasm: A New Health System for the 21st Century. Washington, DC: National Academies Press.

International Council of Nurses. 2006. The Global Nursing Shortage: Priority Areas for Intervention. Geneva: ICN.

———. 2002. Workforce Forum. Available at www.icn.ch.forum2002over view.pdf (accessed August 8, 2008).

International Labour Office. 2006. Migration of Health Workers: Country Case Study Philippines. Geneva: ILO.

International Longevity Center and Schmieding Center for Senior Health and Education Taskforce. 2007. Caregiving in America. The Caregiving Project for Older Americans. New York: International Longevity Center.

International Organization for Migration. 2010. The Role of Migrant Care Workers in Ageing Societies: Report on Research Findings in the United Kingdom, Ireland, and the United States. Geneva: IOM.

———. 2005. World Migration Report: Costs and Benefits of International Migration. Geneva: IOM.

Iredale, R. 2005. Gender immigration policies and accreditation: Valuing the skills of professional women emigrants. *Geoforum* 36: 155–66.

Jamaican Ministry of Health: Nursing Division. 2004. Demand for Registered Nurses Based on Existing Care. Kingston, Jamaica: Ministry of Health.

Jenson, J., and Jacobzone, S. 2000. Care Allowances for the Frail Elderly and Their Impact on Women Caregivers. OECD Labour Market and Social Policy Occasional Papers, no. 41. Paris: OECD.

Johnson, R. W., and Lo Sasso, A. T. 2006. The impact of elder care on women's labor supply at midlife. *Inquiry* 43 (3): 195–210.

Johnson, R. W., Lo Sasso, A. T., Toohey, D., and Wiener, J. M. 2007. Meeting the Long-term Care Needs of the Baby Boomers: How Changing Families Will Affect Paid Helpers and Institutions. Washington, DC: Urban Institute.

Johnson, R. W., Lo Sasso, A. T., and Wiener, J. M. 2006. A Profile of Frail Older Americans and Their Caregivers. Washington, DC: Urban Institute.

Jones, A. 2008. A silent but mighty river: The costs of women's economic migration. *Signs* 33 (4): 761–69.

Jones, A., Bifulco, A. and Gabe, J. 2009. Caribbean nurses migrating to the UK: A gender-focused literature review. *International Nursing Review* 56 (3): 285–90.

Jones, A., Sharpe, J., and Sogren, M. 2004. Children's experiences of separation as a consequence of parental migration. *Caribbean Journal of Social Work* 4 (3): 89–109.

Kaiser Family Foundation. 2010a. The US Global Health Initiative: Key Issues. Available at www.kff.org (accessed November 4, 2010).

———. 2010b. US Participation in International Health Treaties, Commitments, Partnerships, and Other Agreements. Available at www.kff.org (accessed November 4, 2010).

Kane, R. A. 2003. Human resources for long-term care: Lessons from the United States. Key Policy Issues in Long-Term Care. Geneva: WHO, chapter 6.

Kapur, D. 2003. Remittances: The new development mantra? Paper presented at the G-24 Technical Group Meeting, Boston, MA, August 25, Harvard University with the Center for Global Development.

Kassner, E., Reinhard, S., Fox-Grage, W., Houser, A., Accuis, J., et al. 2008. A Balancing Act: State Long-term Care Reform. Washington, DC: AARP Public Policy Institute.

Kelly, P., and D'Addario, S. 2008. "Filipinos are very strongly into medical stuff": Labour market segmentation in Toronto, Canada. In J. Connell, ed., The International Migration of Health Workers. New York: Routledge.

Khadria, B. 2007. International nurse recruitment in India. *Health Services Research* 42 (3): 1429–36.

Kim, N. 2007. The impact of remittances on labor supply: The case of Jamaica. World Bank Policy Research Working Paper 4120 (February).

Kingma, M. 2006. Nurses on the Move: Migration and the Global Health Care Economy. New York: ILR Press.

Kingsland, S. 1995. Modeling Nature: Episodes in the History of Population Ecology. Chicago: University of Chicago Press.

Kittay, E. F. 2002. Can contractualism justify state-supported long-term care policies? Or, I'd rather be some mother's child. A reply to Nussbaum and Daniels. In Ethical Choices in Long-term Care: What Does Justice Require? Geneva: WHO.

———. 2001. A feminist public ethic of care meets the new communitarian family policy. *Ethics* 111 (3): 523–47.

Kofman, E. 2007. Gendered migrations: Livelihoods and entitlements in European welfare regimes. In N. Piper, ed., New Perspectives on Gender and Migration: Livelihoods, Rights, and Entitlement. London: Routledge.

Kofman, E., and Raghuram, P. 2006. Gender and global labour migrations: Incorporating skilled workers. *Antipode* 38 (2): 282–303.

Kofman, E., Phizacklea, A., Raghuram, P., and Sales, R. 2000. Gender and International Migration in Europe: Employment, Welfare and Politics. London: Routledge.

Kovner, C. T., Mezey, M., and Harrington, C. 2002. Who cares for older adults? Workforce implications of an aging society. *Health Affairs* 21 (5): 78–89.

Kramarow, E., Lubitz, J., Lentzner, H., and Gorina, Y. 2007. Trends in the health of older Americans, 1970–2005. *Health Affairs* 26 (5): 1417–25.

Krieger, N. 2001. A glossary of social epidemiology. *Journal of Epidemiology and Community Health* 55: 693–700.

Kuenyehia, A. 1994. The impact of structural adjustment programs on women's human international rights: The example of Ghana. In R. Cook, ed., Human Rights of Women: National and International Perspectives. Philadelphia: University of Pennsylvania Press.

Kunz, R. 2009. The global remittance trend under threat? Paper presented at the International Studies Association, New York, New York, February 13.

Kurasawa, F. 2007. The Work of Global Justice: Human Rights as Practices. Cambridge: Cambridge University Press.

Lairap, J. 2009. Migration, remittances, and microfinance: The impact of increasing feminization of migration, remittances, and microfinance on African women. Paper presented at the International Studies Association, New York, New York, February 13.

Lawlor, E. 2007. Imagining Medicare's next generation. *Public Policy and Aging Report* 16 (3): 3–8.

Le, C. N. 2010. The 1965 Immigration Act. Asian nation: The landscape of Asian America. Available at www.asian-nation.org/1965-immigration -act.shtml (accessed August 8, 2010).

Lethbridge, J. 2004. Brain drain: Re-thinking allocation. *Bulletin of the World Health Organization* 82 (8): 623.

Leutz, W. N. 2007. Immigration and the elderly: Foreign-born workers in long-term care. *Immigration Policy in Focus* 5 (12): 1–11.

Levenson, S. A., and Saffel, D. 2007. The consulting pharmacist and the physician in the nursing home: Roles, relationships, and a recipe for success. *Consultant Pharmacist* 22 (1): 71–82.

Levine, C. 1999. Home sweet hospital: The nature and limits of private responsibilities for home health care. *Journal of Aging Health* 11 (3): 341–59.

———. 1998. Rough Crossings: Family Caregivers' Odysseys through the Health Care System. New York: United Hospital Fund.

Levin, C., Albert, S. M., Hokenstad, A., Halper, D. E., Hart, A. Y., and Gould, D. A. 2006. "This case is closed": Family caregivers and the termination of home health care services for stroke patients. *Milbank Quarterly* 84 (2): 305–31.

Lilly, M. B., Laporte, A., and Coyte, P. C. 2007. Labor market work and home care's unpaid caregivers: A systematic review of labor force participation rates, predictors of labor market withdrawal, and hours of work. *Milbank Quarterly* 85 (4): 641–90.

Lopez-Ortega, M., Matarazzo, C., and Nigenda, G. 2007. Household care for the elderly and the ill in Mexico: An analysis from a gender perspective. In L. Reichenbach, ed., Exploring the Gender Dimensions of the Global Health Workforce. Cambridge, MA: Global Equity Initiative, Harvard University.

Lorenzo, F. M., Galvez-Tan, J., Icamina, K., and Javier, L. 2007. Nurse migration from a source country perspective: Philippine country case Study. *Health Services Research* 42 (3 Pt. 2): 1406–18.

Lorenzo, F. M. E., and Dela, F. R. J., Paraso, G. R., Villegas, S., Issac, C., Yabes, J., Trinidad, F., Fernando, G., and Atienza, J. 2005. Migration of Health Workers: Country Case Study. Institute of Health Policy and Development Studies: National Institute of Health.

Loriaux, S. 2006. Rethinking beneficence and distributive justice in a globalising world. *Global Society* 20 (3): 251–65.

Lowell, B. L., and Findlay, A. 2002. Migration of Highly Skilled Persons from Developing Countries: Impact and Policy Responses—Synthesis Report. International Migration Papers 44. Geneva: ILO.

Lynch, S., Lethola, P., and Ford N. 2008. International nurse migration and HIV/AIDS, Reply. *JAMA* 300 (9): 1024.

Maas, M. L., and Buckwalter, K. C. 2006. Proving quality care in assisted living facilities: Recommendations for enhanced staffing and staff training. *Journal of Gerontological Nursing* 32 (11): 14–22.

McCann, J. J., Hebert, L. E., Beckett, L. A., Morris, P. A., Scherr, P. A., and Evans, D. A. 2000. Comparison of informal caregiving by black and white older adults in a community population. *Journal of the American Geriatrics Society* 48: 1612–17.

McGilton, K. S., Hall, L. M., Wodchis, W. P., and Petroz, U. 2007. Supervisory support, job stress, and job satisfaction among long-term care nursing staff. *Journal of Nursing Administration* 37 (7–8): 366–72.

McKay, D. 2004. Performing identities, creating cultures of circulation: Filipina migrants between home and abroad. Paper presented at Asian Studies Association of Australia, Canberra, June 29.

———. 2003. Cultivating new local futures: Remittance economies and land-use patterns in Ifugao, Philippines. *Journal of Southeast Asian Studies* 34 (2): 285–306.

Mackintosh, M., and Koivusalo, M. 2005. Health systems and commercialization: In search of good sense. In Commercialization of Health Care: Global and Local Dynamics and Policy Responses. UNRISD, Geneva: Palgrave Macmillan.

Mackintosh, M., Mensah, K., and Rowson, M. 2006. Aid, restitution, and fiscal redistribution in health care: Implications of health professionals' migration. *Journal of International Development* 18: 757–70.

Makina, A. 2009. Caring for people with HIV: State policies and their dependence on women's unpaid work. *Gender and Development* 17 (2): 309–19.

Manzano, G. 2005. Quantitative Dimensions: Professional Manpower

Demand, Supply, and Migration Trends. Preliminary draft, Philippines Country Report.

Martin, P. 2005. Merchants of Labour: Agents of the Evolving Migration Infrastructure. Geneva: International Institute for Labour Studies Discussion Paper DP/158/2005.

Martin, S., Lowell, B. L., Gozdziak, E. M., Bump, M., and Breeding, M. E. 2009. The Role of Migrant Care Workers in Aging Societies: Report on Research Findings in the United States. Washington, DC: Institute for the Study of International Migration, Georgetown University.

Massey, D. 2006. Space, time, and political responsibility in the midst of global inequality. *Erdkunde* 60 (2): 89–95.

———. 2004. Geographies of responsibility. *Geografiska Annnaler* 86: 5–18.

Matsuno, A. 2009. Nurse Migration: The Asian perspective. ILO/EU Asian Programme on the Governance of Labour Migration Technical Note.

MedPAC. 2006a. Report to the Congress: Increasing the Value of Medicare. Washington, DC: MedPAC.

———. 2006b. Report to the Congress: Promoting Greater Efficiency in Medicare. Washington, DC: MedPAC.

Meghani, Z., and Eckenwiler, L. 2009. Care for the caregivers? Transnational justice and undocumented non-citizen care workers. *International Journal of Feminist Approaches to Bioethics* 2 (1): 77–101.

Messing, K., and Östlin, P. 2006. Gender Equality, Work, and Health: A Review of the Evidence. Geneva: WHO.

MetLife Mature Market Institute. 2009. MetLife Study of Employee Benefits Trends: Findings from the National Survey of Employers and Employees. Available at www.MatureMarketInstitute.com (accessed August 4, 2010).

MetLife Mature Market Institute and National Alliance for Caregiving. 2006. The MetLife Caregiving Cost Study: Productivity Losses to U.S. Business. Available at www.MatureMarketInstitute.com (accessed August 4, 2010).

MetLife Mature Market Institute, National Alliance for Caregiving, and the National Center on Women and Aging. 1999. The MetLife Juggling Act Study: Balancing Caregiving with Work and the Costs Involved. Available at www.MatureMarketInstitute.com (accessed August 4, 2010).

MetLife Mature Market Institute and University of Pittsburgh Institute on Aging. 2010. The MetLife Study of Working Caregivers and Employer Health Care Costs: New Insights and Innovations for Reducing Health

Care Costs for Employers. Available at www.MatureMarketInstitute .com (accessed August 4, 2010).

Miller, E. A., Booth, M., and Mor, V. 2008. Assessing experts' views of the future of long-term care. *Research on Aging* 30 (4): 450–73.

Miller, E. A., and Weissert, W. G. 2000. Predicting elderly people's risk for nursing home placement, hospitalization, functional impairment and mortality: A synthesis. *Medical Care Research and Review* 57 (3): 259–97.

Miller, S. C. 2009. Moral injury and relational harm: Analyzing rape in Darfur. *Journal of Social Philosophy* 40 (4): 504–23.

Mittelman, M. S., Haley, W. E., Clay, O. J., and Roth, D. L. 2006. Improving caregiver well-being delays nursing home placement of patients with Alzheimer's disease. *Neurology* 67 (9): 1592–99.

Moghadam, V. M. 1999. Gender and the global economy. In M. M. Ferree, J. Lorber, and B. B. Hess, eds., Revisioning Gender. Lanham, MD: Alta Mira Press.

Mohanty, C. 2003. Feminism without Borders. Durham, NC: Duke University Press.

Montgomery, R. J. V., Holley, L., Deichert, J., Kosloski, K. D. 2005. A profile of home care workers from the 2000 census: How it changes what we know. *Gerontologist* 45 (5): 593–600.

National Alliance for Caregiving and AARP. 2004. Caregiving in the U.S. Available at www.caregiving.org/data/04finalreport.pdf (accessed July 7, 2008).

National Commission on Nursing Workforce for Long-Term Care. 2005. Act Now for Your Tomorrow. National Commission on Nursing Workforce for Long-Term Care: Washington, DC.

National Council of State Boards of Nursing. 2008. Knowledge of Newly Licensed Registered Nurses Survey. Research Brief no. 37.

National Family Caregivers Association and Family Caregiver Alliance. 2006. Prevalence, hours, and economic value of family caregiving. Updated state-by-state analysis of 2004 national estimates. Available at www.caregiver.org/caregiver/jsp/content/pdf/State_Caregiving_Data_Arno_20061107.pdf (accessed July 7, 2008).

National Partnership for Women and Families. 2007. Fact sheet: Bush changes to FMLA. Washington, DC: National Partnership for Women and Families.

Navaie-Waliser, M., Feldman, P. H., Gould, D. A., Levine, C., Kuerbis,

A. N., and Donelan, K. 2002. When the caregiver needs care: The plight of vulnerable caregivers. *American Journal of Public Health* 92 (3): 409–13.

National Commission for Quality Long-term Care. 2007. From Isolation to Integration: Recommendations to Improve Quality in Long-term Care. Washington, DC: National Commission for Quality Long-term Care.

Needleman, J., Buerhaus, P., Mattke, S., Stewart, M., and Zelevinsky, K. 2002. Nurse-staffing levels and quality of care in hospitals. *New England Journal of Medicine* 346 (22): 1715–22.

Nelson, J. L. 2002. Just expectations: Family caregivers, practical identities, and social justice in the provision of health care. In R. Rhodes, M. P. Battin, and A. Silvers, eds., Medicine and Social Justice: Essays on the Distribution of Health Care. New York: Oxford University Press.

Newcomer, R., and Scherzer, T. 2006. Who counts? On (not) counting occupational injuries in home care. Paper presented at the American Public Health Association, November 7, Boston, MA.

New York Times, 2003. Editorial, July 8: Is home care really working?

Norrish, B., and Rundall, T. 2001. Hospital re-structuring and the work of registered nurses. *Milbank Quarterly* 79 (1): 55–79.

Nowak, J. 2009. Gendered perceptions of migration among skilled female Ghanaian nurses. *Gender and Development* 17 (2): 269–80.

Nussbaum, M. C. 2006. Frontiers of Justice: Disability, Nationality, Species Membership. Cambridge, MA: Belknap Press of Harvard University Press.

Nurse-ing NRI dreams, they flock to Kochi (n.a.). 2003. Available at www.thehindu.com/thehindu/mp/2003/09/29/2003092900320100.htm (accessed April 20, 2010).

Nynäs, P. 2008. Global vagabonds, place, and the self: The existential dimension of mobility. In S. Bergmann, T. Hoff, and T. Sager, eds., Spaces of Mobility: The Planning, Ethics, Engineering, and Religion of Human Motion. London: Equinox.

Ogden, J., Esim, S., and Grown, C. 2006. Expanding the care continuum for HIV/AIDS: Bringing carers into focus. *Health Policy and Planning* 21 (5): 333–42.

O'Neill, O. 2004. Global justice: Whose obligations? In D. K. Chatterjee, ed., The Ethics of Assistance: Morality and the Distant Needy. Cambridge: Cambridge University Press.

————. 2000. Bounds of Justice. Cambridge: Cambridge University Press.

Ong, A. 2009. A bio-cartography: Maids, neo-slavery, and NGOs. In S. Benhabib and J. Resnik, eds., Migrations and Mobilities: Citizenship, Borders, and Gender. New York: New York University Press.

Organisation for Economic Cooperation and Development (OECD). 2008. International mobility of health workers: Interdependency and ethical challenges. In The Looming Crisis in the Health Workforce: How Can OECD Countries Respond? Paris: OECD.

————. 2005. Ensuring Quality Long-term Care for Older People. OECD Policy Brief. Paris: OECD.

————. 2002. International Migration of Physicians and Nurses: Causes, Consequences, and Health Policy Implications. Paris: OECD.

Packer, C., Labonté, R., and Runnels, V. 2009. Globalization and the cross-border flow of health workers. In R. Labonté, T. Schrecker, C. Packer, and V. Runnels, eds., Globalization and Health: Pathways, Evidence and Policy. New York: Routledge.

Packer, C., Labonté R., and Spitzer, D. (for the WHO Commission on Social Determinants of Health). 2007. Globalization and the Health Worker Crisis. Globalization and Health Knowledge Network Research Papers.

Page, J., and Plaza, S. 2006. Migration remittances and development: A review of global evidence. *Journal of African Economies* 2: 245–336.

Palaganas, E. 2010. Personal communication, November 1.

Pallasmaa, J. 2008. Existential homelessness: Placelessness and nostalgia. In T. P. Uteng and T. Creswell, eds., The Age of Mobility: Gendered Mobilities. Aldershot, Hampshire, England: Ashgate.

Pan American Health Organization. 2005. Nursing shortage threatens health care. *PAHO Today*. Washington, DC: PAHO.

————. 2004a. Profile of the older people of Latin America and the Caribbean. Press Release, January 13. Washington, DC: PAHO.

————. 2004b. The state of aging and health in Latin America and the Caribbean. Press release, January 13. Washington, DC: PAHO.

————. 2004c. PAHO calls for action plan to deal with senior boom in the Americas. Washington, DC: PAHO.

————. 2004d. Women bear burden of home care. Washington, DC: PAHO.

Paraprofessional Health Institute (PHI). 2011. Who are direct care workers? Bronx, NY: PHI.

————. 2010a. Occupational projections for direct care workers, 2008–2018. Bronx, NY: PHI.

———. 2010b. State chart book on wages for personal and home care aides, 1999–2009. Bronx, NY: PHI.

———. 2003. Training Quality Home Care Workers. Bronx, NY: National Clearinghouse on the Direct Care Workforce.

———. 2001. Direct Care Workers: The Unnecessary Crisis in Long-Term Care. Washington, DC: Aspen Institute.

Parekh, S. 2008. Care and human rights in a globalized world. *Southern Journal of Philosophy* 46: 104–10.

Parreñas, R. S. 2006. Understanding the backlash: Why transnational migrant families are considered the "wrong kind of family" in the Philippines. Unpublished manuscript.

———. 2005. Children of Global Migration: Transnational Families and Gendered Woes. Stanford, CA: Stanford University Press.

———. 2001a. Servants of Globalization: Women, Migration, and Domestic Work. Stanford, CA: Stanford University Press.

———. 2001b. Transgressing the nation state: The partial citizenship and "imagined (global) community" of migrant Filipina domestic workers. *Signs* 26 (4): 1129–54.

———. 2000. Migrant Filipina domestic workers and the international division of reproductive labour. *Gender and Society* 14 (4): 560–81.

Parry, C., Coleman, E. A., Smith, J. D., Frank, J., and Kramer, A. M. 2003. The care transitions intervention: A patient-centered approach to ensuring effective transfers between sites of geriatric care. *Home Health Services Quarterly* 22 (3): 1–17.

Patterson, C. 2009. Citizenship and gender in the ancient world: The experience of Athens and Rome. In S. Benhabib and J. Resnik, eds., Migrations and Mobilities: Citizenship, Borders, and Gender. New York: New York University Press.

Pavalko, E. K., and Henderson, K. A. 2006. Combining care work and paid work. *Research on Aging* 28 (3): 359–74.

Pavalko, E. K., Henderson, K. A., and Cott, A. 2008. Workplace policies and caregiving. In M. E. Szinovacz and A. Davey, eds., Caregiving Contexts: Cultural, Familial, and Societal Expectations. New York: Springer.

Pear, R. 2008. Violations reported at 94% of nursing homes. *New York Times*, September 30.

———. 2006. Nursing home inspections miss violations, report says. *New York Times*, January 16.

People's Health Movement. 2005. Global Health Watch: An Alternative Health Report. Medact and Global Equity Guage Alliance. London: Zed Books.

Percot, M. 2006. Indian nurses in the Gulf: Two generations of female migration. *South Asia Research* 26: 41–62.

Pessar, P. R. 2005. Women, Gender, and International Migration across and beyond the Americas: Inequalities and Limited Empowerment. Expert Group Meeting on International Migration and Development in Latin America and the Caribbean. Population Division, Department of Economic and Social Affairs, United Nations Secretariat. Mexico City, November 30–December 2. UN/POP/EGM-MIG/2005/08.

Pessar, P. R., and Mahler, S. J. 2003. Transnational migration: Bringing gender in. *IMR* 37 (3): 812–46.

Philippine Overseas Employment Administration. 2004. Deployed new hire land-based workers by sex, 1992–2002. Available at www.poea .gov.ph/html/statistics.html (accessed May 25, 2009).

Pickett, S. T. A., Kolasa, J., and Jones, C. G. 2007. Ecological Understanding: The Nature of Theory and the Theory of Nature. Boston: Elsevier.

Picone, G., Wilson, R. M., and Chou, S. 2003. Analysis of hospital length of stay and discharge destination using hazard functions with unmeasured heterogeneity. *Health Economics* 12 (12): 1021–34.

Pienkos, A. 2006. Caribbean Labor Migration: Minimizing Losses and Optimizing Benefits. Port of Spain, Trinidad and Tobago: ILO.

Pleis, J. R., and Lethbridge-Cejku, M. 2007. Summary Health Statistics for U.S. Adults: National Health Interview Survey, 2006. Hyattsville, MD: National Center for Health Statistics.

Pinquart, M., and Sørenson, S. 2005. Ethnic differences in stressors, resources, and psychological outcomes of family caregiving: A meta analysis. *Gerontologist* 45: 90–106.

———. 2003. Differences between caregivers and non-caregivers in psychological health and physical health: A meta-analysis. *Psychology and Aging* 18 (2): 250–67.

Piper, N. 2005. Gender and migration. Paper prepared for the Policy Analysis and Research Programme of the Global Commission on International Migration. Geneva: Global Commission on International Migration.

Pittman, P., Folsom, A., Bass, E., and Leonhardy, K. 2007. U.S.-Based International Nurse Recruitment: Structure and Practices of a Burgeoning Industry. Washington, DC: Academy Health.

Pogge, T. 2005. Real world justice. *Journal of Ethics* 9: 29–53.

———. 2004. Relational conceptions of justice: Responsibilities for health outcomes. In S. Anand, F. Peter, and A. Sen, eds., Public Health Ethics and Equity. New York: Oxford University Press.

Polsky, D., Ross, S. J., Brush, B. L., and Sochalski, J. 2007. Trends in characteristics and country of origin among foreign-trained nurses in the United States, 1990 and 2000. *American Journal of Public Health* 97 (5): 895–99.

Polverini, F., and Lamura, G. 2004. Labour Supply in Care Services. National Report on Italy. Dublin: European Foundation for the Improvement of Living and Working Conditions.

Pond, B., and McPake B. 2006. The health migration crisis: The role of four Organisation for Economic Cooperation and Development countries. *Lancet* 6736: 68346–53.

Priester, R., and Reinardy, J. R. 2003. Recruiting immigrants for long-term care nursing positions. *Journal of Aging and Social Policy* 15 (4): 1–19.

Purkayastha, B. 2005. Skilled migration and cumulative disadvantage: the case of highly qualified Asian Indian immigrant women in the United States. *Geoforum* 36: 181–96.

Rafferty, A. M. 2005. The seductions of history and the nursing diaspora. *Health and History* 7 (2): 2–16.

Raghuram, P. 2009. Caring about "brain drain" migration in a postcolonial world. *Geoforum* 40: 25–33.

Raghuram, P., and Kofman, E. 2004. Out of Asia: Skilling, re-skilling, and de-skilling of female migrant workers. *Women's Studies International Forum* 27 (2): 95–100.

Raghuram, P., Madge, C., and Noxolo. P. 2009. Rethinking responsibility and care for a postcolonial world. *Geoforum* 40: 5–13.

Ramirez, C., M. G. Dominguez, and J. M. Morais. 2005. Crossing Borders: Remittances, Gender and Development. Santo Domingo: INSTRAW.

Ramji, V. 2002. Income security and hidden care issues: Female careworkers emigrating from Kerala to the Middle East. In Bien Conference Papers of the Infocus Programme of Socio-Economic Security. Geneva: ILO.

Rapoport, H., and Docquier, F. 2005. The Economics of Migrants' Remittances. IZA Discussion Paper 1531.

Redfoot, D., and Houser, A. 2005. "We Shall Travel On": Quality of Care,

Economic Development, and the International Migration of Long-term Care Workers. Washington, DC: AARP Public Policy Institute.

Reichenbach, L. 2007. Exploring the Gender Dimensions of the Global Health Workforce. Cambridge, MA: Global Equity Initiative, Harvard University.

Reinhard, S. C., and Reinhard, T. 2006. Scanning the field: Nursing management and leadership in long-term care. Washington, DC: Institute for the Future of Aging Services.

Reinhard, S. C., and Young, H. M. 2009. The nursing workforce in long-term care. *Nursing Clinics of North America* 44: 161–68.

Richards, P. 2005. Exodus of nurses costs region millions. IPS Inter Press Service News Agency, April 6. Available at www.ipsnews.net/print .asp?idnews=28182 (accessed March 19, 2010).

Robinson, F. 2006. Ethical globalization? States, corporations, and the ethics of care. In M. E. Hammington and D. C. Miller, eds., Socializing Care. Lanham, MD: Rowman & Littlefield.

Rodriguez, R. M. 2008. The labor brokerage state and the globalization of Filipina care workers. *Signs* 33: 794–99.

Romero, M. 2006. Unraveling privilege: Workers' children and the hidden costs of paid childcare. In M. K. Zimmerman, J. S. Litt, and C. E. Bose, eds., Global Dimensions of Gender and Carework. Stanford, CA: Stanford University Press.

Rosenfeld, P. 2007. Workplace practices for retaining older hospital nurses: Implications from a study of nurses with eldercare responsibilities. *Policy, Politics, and Nursing Practice* 8 (2): 120–29.

Royal College of Nursing. 2007. Holding On: Nurses' Employment and Morale in 2007. London: Royal College of Nursing.

Ruger, J. P. 2006. Ethics and governance of heath inequalities. *Journal of Epidemiology and Community Health* 60: 998–1002.

Safri, M., and Graham, J. 2010. The global household: Toward a feminist post-capitalist international political economy. *Signs* 36 (1): 99–125.

Salmon, M. E., Yan, J., Hewitt, H., and Guisinger, V. 2007. Managed migration: The Caribbean approach to addressing nursing services capacity. *Health Services Research* 42 (3, part 2): 1354–72.

Sanders, R. S. 2005. Turning Caribbean migration to advantage. Commentary. Caribbean Net News. Available at www.caribbeanneatnews.com (accessed June 12, 2009).

Sassen, S. 2002a. Global cities and survival circuits. In B. Ehrenreich and A. R. Hochschild, eds., Global Woman: Nannies, Maids, and Sex Workers in the New Economy. New York: Henry Holt.

———. 2002b. Women's burden: Counter-geographies of globalization and the feminization of survival. Nordic Journal of International Law 71 (2): 255–74.

———. 2000. Cities in a World Economy. Thousand Oaks, CA: Pine Forge Press.

SCAN Foundation. 2010. A summary of the Patient Protection and Affordable Care Act and Modifications by the Health Care and Education Reconciliation Act of 2010.

Scanlon, W. J. 2001. Nursing Workforce: Recruitment and Retention of Nurses and Nurse Aides Is a Growing Concern, Report no. GAO-01-750T. Washington, DC: US General Accounting Office (GAO).

Schild, V. 2007. Empowering "consumer-citizens" or governing female subjects? The institutionalization of "self-development" in the Chilean social policy field. Journal of Consumer Culture 7 (2): 179–203.

Schmalzbauer, L. 2004. Searching for wages and mothering from afar: The case of Honduran transnational families. Journal of Marriage and Family 66: 1317–31.

Schrecker, T. 2008. Denaturalizing scarcity: a strategy of enquiry for public-health ethics. Bulletin of the World Health Organization 86 (8): 600–605.

Schulz, R., and Beach, S. R. 1999. Caregiving as a risk factor for mortality: The caregiver health effects study. JAMA 282 (23): 2215.

Schwenken, H. 2008. Beautiful victims and sacrificing heroines: Exploring the role of gender knowledge in migration policies. Signs 33 (4): 770–76.

Seavey, D. 2007. Testimony before the House Committee on Education and Labor, Subcommittee on Workforce Protections, Written Statement. Washington, DC, October 25.

Sevenhuijsen, S., Bozalek, V., Gouws, A., and Minnaar-McDonald, M. 2006. South African welfare policy. An analysis through the network of care. In M. E. Hamington, and D. C. Miller, eds., Socializing Care. Lanham, MD: Rowman & Littlefield.

Shrestha, L. B. 2000. Population aging in developing countries. Health Affairs 19 (3): 204–12.

Skjold, S. 2007. The gender dimensions of unpaid work in health care. In L. Reichenbach, ed., Exploring the Gender Dimensions of the Global Health Workforce. Cambridge, MA: Global Equity Initiative, Harvard University.

Sørenson, N. N. 2005a. Narratives of longing, belonging, and caring in the Dominican diaspora. In J. Besson and K. F. Olwig, eds., Caribbean Narratives of Belonging: Fields of Relations, Sites of Identity. Thailand: Macmillan Caribbean.

———. 2005b. The development dimension of migrant remittances: Towards a gendered typology. Paper presented at the International Forum on Remittances, Washington, DC, June 28–30.

———. 2004. The development dimension of migrant remittances. IOM Working Paper Series no. 1, Department of Migration Policy, Research, and Communications. Geneva: IOM.

Spatafora, N. 2005. Two current issues facing developing countries. In World Economic Outlook: A Survey by the Staff of the IMF. Washington, DC: IMF.

Stacey, C. L. 2005. Finding dignity in dirty work: The constraints and rewards of low-wage home care labour. Sociology of Health and Illness 27 (6): 831–54.

Stark, O., Helmenstein, C., and Prskawetz, A. 1998. Human capital depletion, human capital formation, and migration: A blessing or a curse? Economics Letters 60: 363–67.

Stearns, S. C., and D'Arcy, L. P. 2008. Staying the course: Facility and profession retention among nursing assistants in nursing homes. Journals of Gerontology: Social Sciences 63B: S113–S121.

Steinbrook, R. 2002. Nursing in the crossfire. New England Journal of Medicine 346 (22): 1757–66.

Stilwell, B., Diallo, K., Zurn, P., Vujicic, M., Adams, O., and Dal Poz, M. 2004. Migration of health care workers from developing countries: Strategic approaches to its management. Bulletin of the World Health Organization 82: 595–600.

Stone, R. 2000. Long-term Care for the Elderly with Disbilities: Current Policy, Emerging Trends, and Implications for the 21st Century. New York: Milbank Memorial Fund.

Stone, R., and Wiener, J. 2001. Who Will Care for Us?: Addressing the Long-term Care Workforce Crisis. Washington, DC: Urban Institute.

Szlezák, N. A., Bloom, B. R., Jamison, D. T., Keusch, G. T., Michaud, C. M., Moon, S., and Clark, W. C. 2010. The global health system: Actors, norms, and expectations in transition. *PLoS Medicine* 7 (1): 1–4.

Tan, E. 2003. Realities and challenges for the global nursing community. *Philippine Journal of Nursing* 71 (1–2): 8–10.

Thomas, C., R. Hosein, and Yan, J. 2005. Assessing the Export of Nursing Services as a Diversification Option for CARICOM Economies. Caribbean Commission on Health and Development. Georgetown, Guyana: CARICOM.

Thomas, P. 2010. Personal communication, October 17.

———. 2006. The international migration of Indian nurses. *International Nursing Review* 53 (4): 277–83.

Thomas-Hope, E. 2005. Current trends and issues in Caribbean migration. In Regional and International Migration in the Caribbean and Its Impact on Sustainable Development: Compendium on Recent Research on Migration in the Caribbean, Caribbean Expert Group Meeting on Migration, Human Rights and Development in the Caribbean, September.

Tolentino, R. B. 1996. Bodies, letters, catalogs: Filippinas in transnational space. *Social Text* 48 (Autumn): 49–76.

Tronto, J. 2006. Vicious circles of privatized caring. In M. E. Hamington and D. C. Miller, eds., Socializing Care. Lanham, MD: Rowman & Littlefield.

Truong, T. D. 1996. Gender, international migration and social reproduction: Implications for theory, policy, research, and networking. *Asian and Pacific Migration Journal* 5 (1): 27–52.

Tyner, J. A. 2004. Made in the Philippines: Gendered Discourses and The Making of Migrants. London: Routledge.

———. 1996. The gendering of Philippine international labor migration. *Professional Geographer* 48 (4): 405–16.

Uhlenberg, P., and Cheuk, M. 2008. Demographic change and the future of informal caregiving. In M. E. Szinovacz and A. Davey, eds., Caregiving Contexts: Cultural, Familial, and Societal Expectations. New York: Springer.

Ungerson, C. 1997. Social politics and the commodification of care. *Social Politics* (Fall): 362–82.

———. 2004. Whose empowerment and independence? A cross-national perspective on "cash for care" schemes. *Aging and Society* 24: 189–212.

United Nations. 2002. International Migration, 2002. New York: UN.

United Nations Population Fund. 2006. State of World Population 2006: A Passage to Hope: Women and International Migration. New York: UNFPA.

United Nations Population Fund—Caribbean. N.d. Population Ageing. New York: UNFPA.

U.S. Administration on Aging. 2007. 2005 National Ombudsman Reporting System Data Tables. Washington, DC: U.S. Administration on Aging.

———. 2001. Older Adults and Mental Health: Issues and Opportunities. Washington, DC: U.S. Department of Health and Human Services (DHHS).

U.S. Bureau of Labor Statistics (USBLS). 2009. Nonfatal Occupational Injuries and Illnesses Requiring Days Away from Work, 2009. Washington, DC: USBLS.

———. 2007. Occupational employment projections to 2016. *Monthly Labor Review* (November).

U.S. Census Bureau. 2008. Statistical Abstract of the United States: 2008. Washington, DC: U.S. Census Bureau.

U.S. Department of Health and Human Services (DHHS). 2000. The Characteristics of Long-term Care Users. Rockville, MD: Agency for Healthcare Research and Quality.

U.S. Department of Health and Human Services (DHHS) and Health Resources and Services Administration (HRSA). 2004a. Nursing Aides, Home Health Aides, and Related Health Care Occupations: National and Local Workforce Shortages and Associated Data Needs. HRSA: Washington, DC.

———. 2004b. Projected Supply, Demand, and Shortages of Registered Nurses: 2000–2020. Available at http://bhpr.hrsa.gov/healthworkforce/reports/rnproject/report.htm (accessed June 19, 2008).

U.S. Department of Health and Human Services (DHHS) and U.S. Department of Labor (DOL). 2003. The Future Supply of Long-Term Care Workers in Relation to the Aging Baby Boom Generation: Report to Congress. Washington, DC: Office of the Assistant Secretary for Planning and Evaluation.

U.S. Government Accountability Office (GAO). 2005. Nursing Homes: Despite Increased Oversight, Challenges Remain in Ensuring High-Quality Care and Resident Safety (GAO-06-117). Washington, DC: Government Accountability Office.

U.S. Special Committee on Aging. United States Senate (February, 2000). Developments in Aging: 1997 and 1998, vol. 1, Report 106–229. Washington, DC: U.S. Government Printing Office.

Uy-Eviota, E. 1992. The Political Economy of Gender: Women and the Sexual Division of Labour in the Philippines. London: Zed.

Van Eyck, K. 2005. Who Cares? Women Health Workers in the Global Labour Market. Ferney-Voltaire, France: PSI.

———. 2004. Women and International Migration in the Health Sector: Final Report of Public Service International's Participatory Action Research 2003. Ferney-Voltaire, France: PSI.

Vega, E. 2007. Health and aging in Latin America and the Caribbean. In M. Robinson, W. Novelli, C. Pearson, L. Norris, eds., Health and Global Aging. San Francisco: Jossey-Bass.

Vidal, J. P. 1998. The effect of emigration on human capital formation. *Journal of Population Economics* 11: 589–600.

Vitaliano, P. P., Zhang, J., and Scanlan, J. M. 2003. Is caregiving hazardous to one's physical health? A meta analysis. *Psychological Bulletin* 129 (6): 946–72.

von Mering, O. 1996. American culture and long-term care. In R. H. Binstock, L. E. Cluff, and O. von Mering, eds., The Future of Long-Term Care. Baltimore: Johns Hopkins University Press.

Waage, J., Banerji, R., and Campbell, O. 2010. The Millennium Development Goals: A cross-sectoral analysis and principles for goal-setting after 2015. *Lancet* 376: 991–1023.

Wakabayashi, C., and Donato, K. M. 2006. Does caregiving increase poverty among women in later life? Evidence from the Health and Retirement Survey. *Journal of Health and Social Behavior* 47 (3): 258–74.

Waldfogel, J. 2001. Family and Medical Leave: Evidence from the 2000 surveys. *Monthly Labor Review* 124 (9): 17–23.

Waldron, T. 2004. Global positioning. *Johns Hopkins Nursing* 2 (1). Available at www.son.jhmi.edu/JHNmagazine/archive/spring2004/pages/fea_globalpositioning.html (accessed August 9, 2010).

Wegelin-Schuringa, M. 2006. Local responses to HIV/AIDS from a gendered perspective. In A. Van der Kwaak and M. Wegelin-Schuring, eds., Gender, Society and Development, Gender and Health, Policy and Practice, A Global Sourcebook. Amsterdam: KIT, Royal Tropical Institute.

Weinberg, D. B. 2003. Code Green: Money-driven Hospitals and the Dismantling of Nursing. New York: Cornell University Press.

Weinberg, D. B., Lusenhop, R. W., Gittell, J. H., and Kautz, C. M. 2007. Coordination between formal providers and informal caregivers. *Health Care Management Review* 32 (2): 140–49.

Weinberger, M. B. 2007. Population aging: A global overview. In M. Robinson, W. Novelli, C. Pearson, and L. Norris, eds., Global Health and Global Aging. San Francisco: Jossey-Bass.

Wenger, N. S., Solomon, D. H., Roth, C. P., MacLean, C. H., Saliba, D. ... and Shekelle, P. G. 2003. The quality of medical care provided to vulnerable community-dwelling older patients. *Annals of Internal Medicine* 139 (9): 740–47.

Weuve, J. L., Boult, C., and Morishita, L. 2000. The effects of outpatient geriatric management on caregiver burden. *Gerontologist* 40 (4): 429–36.

Wiener, J. M. 2003. The role of informal support in long-term care. In Key Policy Issues in Long-term Care. Geneva: WHO.

Williams, J. C., and Boushey, H. 2010. The Three Faces of Work-Family Conflict. Washington, DC: Center for American Progress and Center for Worklife Law.

Wolff, J. L. 2007. Supporting and Sustaining the Family Caregiver Workforce for Older Americans. Paper commissioned by IOM Committee on the Future Health Care Workforce for Older Americans. Unpublished.

Wolff, J. L., and Kasper, J. D. 2006. Caregivers of frail elders: Updating a national profile. *Gerontologist* 46 (3): 344–56.

Wolff, J. L., Starfield, B., and Anderson, G. 2002. Prevalence, expenditures, and complications of multiple chronic conditions in the elderly. *Archives of Internal Medicine* 162 (20): 2269–76.

World Bank. 2005. Global Economic Prospects 2006: Economic Implications of Remittances and Migration. Washington, DC: World Bank.

———. 2004. Global Economic Finance 2003. Washington, DC: World Bank.

World Health Organization (WHO). 2009. International Long-term Care Initiative. Geneva: WHO.

———. 2008. International Recruitment of Health Personnel: Draft Global Code of Practice. Geneva: WHO.

———. 2006a. Migration of Health Workers. Geneva: WHO.

———. 2006b. What Are the Public Health Implications of Global Ageing? Geneva: WHO.

———. 2006c. World Health Report 2006: Working Together for Health. Geneva: WHO.

———. 2004. Migration of Health Professionals in Six Countries: A Synthesis Report. Brazzaville, South Africa: WHO Regional Office for Africa.

———. 2003. Key Policy Issues in Long-term Care. Geneva: WHO.

———. 2002a. Current and Future Long-term Care Needs: An Analysis Based on the 1990 WHO Study, The Global Burden of Disease. Geneva: WHO.

———. 2002b. Ethical Choices in Long-term Care: What Does Justice Require? Geneva: WHO.

———. 2002c. Lessons for Long-term Care Policy. Geneva: WHO.

———. 2000. World Health Report 2000—Health Systems: Improving Performance. Geneva: WHO.

Xu, Y., and Kwak, C. 2005. Changing faces: Internationally educated nurses in U.S. workforce in long-term care settings. *Home Health Care Management and Practice* 17 (5): 421–23.

Yan, J. 2006. Health services delivery: Reframing policies for global nursing migration in North America: A Caribbean perspective. *Policy, Politics, and Nursing Practice* 7 (3): Supplement 71S–75S.

Yeates, N. 2009. Globalizing Care Economies and Migrant Workers: Explorations in Global Care Chains. Basingstoke, UK: Palgrave Macmillan.

Yoo, B., Bhattacharya, J., McDonald, K., and Garber, A. 2004. Impacts of informal caregiver availability on long-term care expenditures in OECD countries. *Health Services Research* 39 (6): 1971–92.

Young, I. M. 2006. Responsibility and global justice: A social connection model. *Social Philosophy and Policy* 23: 102–30.

———. 2004a. Responsibility and global labor justice. *Journal of Political Philosophy* 12 (4): 365–88.

———. 2004b. Responsibility and structural injustice. Unpublished manuscript.

———. 2000. Inclusion and Democracy. Oxford: Oxford University Press.

———. 1997. Asymmetrical reciprocity: On moral respect, wonder, and enlarged thought. In Dilemmas of Gender, Political Philosophy, and Policy. Princeton: Princeton University Press.

Index

Africa, 15, 33, 64, 97
African Americans, 40
ageism, 19–20, 83
aging. *See* elderly
American Health Care Association, 38
American Hospital Association, 38
American Public Health Association, 97
Asians, 15, 37

becoming and enduring, 11, 79, 82–83, 85, 87, 88, 93, 111n4
body, 5, 78, 79. *See also* embodiment
businesses, 23, 45, 88, 95, 108n3; and family caregivers, 67; and family leave policy, 95–96; responsibilities of, 76, 88. *See also* employers

Canada, 33, 44, 45
capabilities/capacities, 76, 77, 79, 82, 83, 85, 93, 110n3
capitalism, 41, 51, 52, 104
care, 10, 41, 49, 52, 81, 82, 90, 95; cash for, 25, 55, 68; and citizenship, 22; community-based, 19, 94; consumer-directed, 25–26, 68, 108n4; defined, 20; quality of, 8, 9, 16–17, 18, 20, 28, 84, 94. *See also* health care; long-term care
caregivers, 3, 16, 20–21, 58, 101; and financial security, 104; informal/unpaid, 9, 16, 21, 24–25, 26, 54, 95; paid, 9–10, 16, 24–25, 95. *See also* direct care workers; family caregivers; nurses

caregiving, 22, 107n3
care work, 10, 20, 28, 66, 104, 107n3; commodification of, 41; as core public need, 90; and economy, 22; exportation of, 49; by families, 26; and gender, 54, 55; global division of, 50; and justice, 110–111n3; and neoliberalism, 90; paid vs. informal, 25; and race, 40, 41; transnational trade in, 35–36
care workers, 4, 14, 28, 94, 96, 99–100, 101, 102; American need for, 30, 80–81; educated in United States, 10, 32; effects from loss of, 60, 61; emigration of, 7, 35; foreign-educated, 10, 32, 33, 93; global, regional, and local needs of, 90; and globalism, 9, 37; health problems of, 57–58; and home country economies, 35; inadequate training of, 17–18, 24, 68; and injustice, 73, 87; and labor market stratification, 61–62; and planning failures, 8; and poor work conditions, 2; responsibilities to, 89; shortages of, 3, 7, 8, 37, 60–62, 68, 73; and solidarity with family caregivers, 102–4; standards for, 90; transnational flow of, 31–34; undocumented noncitizen, 56, 58; vulnerabilities of, 55–57; work conditions and wages of, 30; working conditions of, 90, 99, 102. *See also* direct care workers; family caregivers; nurses; personal care workers

embodiment, 5, 78, 82, 111n5. *See also* body

emigrants, 2; and class, 42; and downskilling, 53, 62; equal pay, benefits, and worker protection for, 96; families of, 110–111n3; and family leave policy, 95; feminization of labor of, 8; and government policy, 93; growing reliance on, 2–3; health status of, 84; as heroic vs. causing social ills, 52; home countries of, 35, 52, 56, 72, 83; injustice experienced by, 87; and interdependence, 104; and labor laws, 56; from low- and middle-income countries, 31; plight of, 49; and policy, 4; and quality of care, 84; recognition of, 101; remittances from, 58–60; and self-development and self-determination, 83; social and economic vulnerability of, 54; solidarity with family caregivers, 103; and structural injustice, 73; upward and downward mobility of, 53; vulnerabilities of, 55–57; wages and benefits for, 56. *See also* immigrants; migrants

emigration: from Caribbean, 44–46, 64–65; and climate change, 11; and colonialism, 75–76; effects on home country, 60–62; and globalization, 34–36; government dependence on, 35; and health worker shortage, 7; from India, 46–48, 65–66; lost investments from, 61; from Philippines, 35, 41–44, 62–63, 91; reasons for, 10, 35, 41–42, 45, 46; standards for, 90

employers, 50, 72, 108n3; and employees, 89, 102; and family caregivers, 23–24, 26, 67; and family leave policy, 95; and government policy, 93; and preventive foresight, 100; and protection of health systems, 97; responsibilities of, 89. *See also* businesses

equality, 72, 75, 78, 83, 87, 88, 90
European Union, 97

families, 8, 24, 25, 35, 66, 72, 89, 94; and global household, 91–92; and interdependence, 104; and respectful interaction, 101–2

Family Caregiver Alliance, 94

family caregivers, 19; among minority groups, 53; and appreciation of care, 102; and built environment, 96; capacities of, 2–3, 16, 24–25; and changing family profile, 21–22; daughters as, 21; different policy agendas for, 25; diminished capacity of, 28; ecological conception of, 95; effects of caregiving on, 50; and employers, 23–24, 26, 67; and family leave policy, 95; financial assistance to, 26; and fragmentation of health care, 52; and global economic and immigration policy, 8; government support for, 95; and health and labor policy, 8; and health care costs, 7, 8; health problems of, 57–58; hours per month of support by, 21; impoverishment of, 53; initiatives for, 54–55; and injustice, 87; and institutional cost-cutting, 25; loss of benefits by, 53; numbers of available, 21, 22; and paid care workers, 14; as perpetuating inequality, 75; plight of, 9, 20–22; and policy, 2, 4, 93, 94; as primary providers of long-term care, 21; professional sacrifices of, 52, 53; and race and culture, 50; recognition of, 54, 101; responsibilities of, 76; and self-development and self-determination, 83; shortage of, 16; social standing of, 22; solidarity with workers, 102–4; and structural injustice, 73; support and assistance from, 21; women as, 21; working in paid labor force, 7. *See also* caregivers; home care

International Council of Nurses, 43, 97
International Health Partnership, 92
International Labour Organization
   (ILO), 91, 92
international lending bodies, 10,
   70, 71, 88–89, 90, 102. *See also*
   International Monetary Fund; neo-
   liberal economic policies; World
   Bank
International Long-term Care Initia-
   tive, 90
International Monetary Fund (IMF),
   34, 64, 89, 90, 99
intersubjectivity, 80, 81, 84, 103–4

Jamaica, 33, 44, 64, 65
Joint Learning Initiative, 61
justice, 11, 81, 82, 85, 99–100, 102,
   103, 110–11n3; and ecological
   thinking, 7–9, 79; as enablement,
   76–77, 79; and family leave policy,
   95; global, 3, 7–9, 77, 81, 84,
   99–100; and well-being and flourishing, 84. *See also* injustice

labor policy, 10, 23–24, 29, 56
Long Island Care at Home, Ltd. v.
   Coke, 29
long-term care, 41; access to, 72; and
   biomedical model, 17; care worker
   shortages in, 68; complexity and
   cost of, 28; comprehensive and
   coordinated government policy
   for, 93; and consumer-directed
   care, 26; decentralization of, 19;
   defined, 15; and ecological thinking, 49, 70; emigrant workers in,
   32, 33, 63; and family caregivers, 21, 22; funding for, 16; and
   future, 85–86; in global context,
   3, 31, 39, 49, 76; informalization and privatization of, 19, 31;
   and institutional dysfunction,
   16–17; interconnected concerns
   in, 8; and justice, 68–69, 71–74,
   76, 81, 98–99; and Medicaid,
   19; and medical specialties, 18,

24; and Medicare, 19; movement
   from hospital to, 18; and nationalist focus, 9, 74; need for, 2, 3,
   9, 13–14, 15, 90; and neoliberal
   economic policies, 55; policy for,
   2, 3, 11, 74, 83; population of,
   22; principles for, 90; problems
   with, 2, 7, 15, 16–17; protection
   of elderly in, 91; quality of, 2,
   8–9, 67, 68; restructuring for, 95;
   undocumented immigrants in, 38;
   working conditions in, 101; and
   world lending institutions, 90. *See
   also* care; nursing homes
low- and middle-income countries,
   3, 10, 15, 31, 68, 81, 85, 96, 105.
   See also developing countries;
   global South; source countries

mail-order brides, 50–51
managed care, 29, 32
Marcos, Ferdinand, 43
McKinley, William, 62
Medicaid, 19, 58, 94
Medicare, 19, 94
Merck Institute of Aging and Health,
   91
migrants, 2, 10, 55, 85, 89, 91
migration, 31–34, 38, 44, 46, 59,
   64, 65, 89; and absence of health
   workers, 110–11n3; adverse effects
   from, 60, 61; and global household, 92; trends in, 32–33; and
   WHO, 90–91; by women, 39, 60.
   See also emigration
Milbank Memorial Fund, 90
military, 42, 50
Millennium Development Goals
   (MDGs), 92
missionary, 42
Money Follows the Person initiative,
   25

National Center for Assisted Living,
   38
National Commission for Quality
   Long-term Care (NCQLTC), 8

National Family Caregiver Support Program (NFCSP), 26, 54, 94
nationalism, and migrant workers, 51
neoliberal economic policies, 34, 47, 51, 53, 55, 88, 90. *See also* economies
Nigeria, 33, 65
North America, 33, 46. *See also* Canada; United States
nurse aides, 10, 18, 29, 31, 33
nurses, 2, 59, 89, 108n4; and American immigration policy, 37–38; from Caribbean, 45, 46, 64–65; countries of origin of, 32–33; education of, 10, 17–18, 29, 32, 44, 47, 62–63; effects of loss of, 61; from India, 33, 46–48; integral role of, 61, 94; licensure exam for, 33; from low- and middle-income countries, 31; LPNs, 29, 32, 46; numbers of, 27; from Philippines, 33, 35, 41–44, 62–63; pride vs. distress of, 56; ratio to patients, 42, 63; ratio to population in India, 65–66; reasons for emigrating, 41–42, 46; and recruitment industry, 38–39; RNs, 29, 32, 37–38, 41, 42, 46; shortages of, 7, 8, 30, 68; transnational flow of, 31–34; turnover rates among, 30; wages of, 42; working conditions of, 7, 8, 28–29, 42, 45, 46, 65. *See also* caregivers
nursing homes, 2, 18, 19, 25, 27, 31, 94; quality of, 16, 17; worker turnover rates in, 31. *See also* long-term care

Olmstead v. LC, 28

Pan American Health Organization (PAHO), 91
personal care workers, 10, 18, 28, 31, 46
Philippines, 10, 33, 41–44, 49, 62–63; and American immigra-

tion policy, 37; and education, 44, 47; Office of the Undersecretary for Migrant Workers' Affairs, 43; Overseas Workers Welfare Administration, 43; Philippine Overseas Employment Agency, 43; political economy of, 35; wages in, 42; women from, 50–51
physicians, 17, 32, 63
place-making, ethical, 11, 81, 83
poor people, 19, 42, 45, 49, 52, 59, 64, 75; direct care workers as, 29; and ecological thinking, 70; responsibilities to, 89; and world lending institutions, 90
privileged irresponsibility, 75
public health, 80, 90
public sector, 34, 35, 62, 78, 97, 110–11n3

race, 40–41, 50–52
reciprocity, 78, 100, 103, 104
recruiters, 43, 50, 51, 70, 76, 89, 97, 98–99
recruitment, 8, 44, 45; for-profit, 38, 47, 67, 89, 97; by governments, 35; growth of, 38–39; standards for, 90, 91
relationality, 73, 80, 81, 83, 84, 89, 101, 111n5. *See also* connectedness; interdependence
remittances, 58–60, 63, 64, 109–10n5
respect, for care work and care workers, 28, 29
responsibility, 3, 10–11, 78, 85–86, 100, 112n1; assignment of, 85, 88–99; and ecological thinking, 70–71, 81; for equal becoming and enduring, 87, 93; of global actors and institutions, 88; for global justice, 81; global scope of, 74–76; of governments, 93; of international lending bodies, 88; and intersubjectivity, 80; liability conception of, 110n1; networks of, 82; of

Urban Institute, Retirement Project, 14

wages/benefits/income, 42, 45, 46, 67, 94, 102; of direct care workers, 29–30; of emigrants, 40, 63; and immigration policy, 37; and justice, 96, 102; and recruiting, 48; for undocumented noncitizens, 56

wealthy countries, 2, 26, 33, 36, 68, 96; citizens of, 104; education for standards of, 62, 98; elderly population in, 15; flow of resources to, 70; need for care workers in, 8, 80; working conditions in, 7. *See also* global North; host countries

women, 21, 25, 58, 60, 65, 91, 92; of color, 40–41; as direct care workers, 27; and ecological thinking, 70; emigrant, 31, 33, 40, 43, 45, 46–47, 50–51, 66; and emigrant labor, 8; exploitation of, 55–57; flexibilization of, 52–53; and gender norms, 39–40; in global economy, 35–36; and global South, 35, 41; illegal immigration

of, 38; and labor policies, 40–41; migration by, 32, 39–40, 60; paid and unpaid labor of, 36; as primary care givers, 35, 40; and race and culture, 50–52; responsibilities of, 62; skilled labor of, 36; social and political positioning of, 54; support for, 26; white, 40–41; in workforce, 21–22. *See also* gender

working conditions: advocacy for fair, 99, 101, 102; in affluent countries, 7; and businesses, 95; and care quality, 8; and Caribbean emigrants, 45; and ecological thinking, 7; in India, 46; as poor, 45, 46, 49, 65; as poor in United States, 2, 28, 29; and solidarity, 104; standards for, 90

workplace, 23–24, 75, 94, 95, 104, 108n3

World Bank, 34, 89–90, 92, 99

World Health Organization (WHO), 9, 60, 88, 90–91, 92, 97

World Trade Organization (WTO), 36, 92

World War II, 43, 44